Untangling the Racism

A Primer for Pediatric Health Professionals

Editors

Maria Trent, MD, MPH, FSAHM, FAAP

Danielle G. Dooley, MD, MPhil, FAAP

Jacqueline Dougé, MD, MPH, FAAP

With a Foreword by Joseph L. Wright, MD, MPH, FAAP

American Academy of Pediatrics

DEDICATED TO THE HEALTH OF ALL CHILDREN®

American Academy of Pediatrics Publishing Staff

Mary Lou White, *Chief Product and Services Officer/SVP, Membership, Marketing, and Publishing*
Mark Grimes, *Vice President, Publishing*
Carrie Peters, *Editor, Professional/Clinical Publishing*
Theresa Wiener, *Production Manager, Clinical and Professional Publications*
Amanda Helmholz, *Medical Copy Editor*
Sara Hoerdeman, *Marketing and Acquisitions Manager, Consumer Products*

Published by the American Academy of Pediatrics
345 Park Blvd
Itasca, IL 60143
Telephone: 630/626-6000
Facsimile: 847/434-8000
www.aap.org

The American Academy of Pediatrics is an organization of 67,000 primary care pediatricians, pediatric medical subspecialists, and pediatric surgical specialists dedicated to the health, safety, and well-being of all infants, children, adolescents, and young adults.

While every effort has been made to ensure the accuracy of this publication, the American Academy of Pediatrics does not guarantee that it is accurate, complete, or without error.

The recommendations in this publication do not indicate an exclusive course of treatment or serve as a standard of medical care. Variations, taking into account individual circumstances, may be appropriate.

Any websites, brand names, products, or manufacturers are mentioned for informational and identification purposes only and do not imply an endorsement by the American Academy of Pediatrics (AAP). The AAP is not responsible for the content of external resources. Information was current at the time of publication.

The publishers have made every effort to trace the copyright holders for borrowed materials. If they have inadvertently overlooked any, they will be pleased to make the necessary arrangements at the first opportunity.

This publication has been developed by the American Academy of Pediatrics. The contributors are expert authorities in the field of pediatrics. No commercial involvement of any kind has been solicited or accepted in the development of the content of this publication. Disclosures: Dr Hoffman disclosed a financial relationship with the National Drowning Prevention Alliance. Dr Navsaria disclosed a Board of Directors relationship with Reach Out and Read. Any relevant disclosures have been mitigated through a process approved by the AAP Board of Directors.

Every effort is made to keep *Untangling the Thread of Racism: A Primer for Pediatric Health Professionals* consistent with the most recent advice and information available from the American Academy of Pediatrics.

Please visit www.aap.org/errata for an up-to-date list of any applicable errata for this publication.

Special discounts are available for bulk purchases of this publication. Email Special Sales at nationalaccounts@aap.org for more information.

Printed in the United States of America

9-504/1023   1 2 3 4 5 6 7 8 9 10
MA1124
ISBN: 978-1-61002-710-6
eBook: 978-1-61002-711-3

Cover and publication design by Peg Mulcahy

Library of Congress Control Number: 2023904273

American Academy of Pediatrics Reviewers

Committee on Adolescence

Committee on Native American Child Health

Council on Children With Disabilities

Council on Environmental Health and Climate Change

Section on Adolescent Health

Section on Lesbian, Gay, Bisexual, and Transgender Health and Wellness

Section on Minority Health, Equity, and Inclusion

Contributors

Editors

Maria Trent, MD, MPH, FSAHM, FAAP
Bloomberg Professor of American Health, Pediatrics, and Nursing
Senior Associate Dean of Diversity and Inclusive Excellence
Director, Division of Adolescent and Young Adult Medicine
Johns Hopkins University
Baltimore, MD

Danielle G. Dooley, MD, MPhil, FAAP
Medical Director, Community Affairs and Population Health
Child Health Advocacy Institute
Children's National Hospital
Associate Professor of Pediatrics
George Washington University School of Medicine and Health Sciences
Washington, DC

Jacqueline Dougé, MD, MPH, FAAP
Assistant Professor of Public Health
Department of Nursing
Hood College
Frederick, MD

Authors

Anisha Abraham, MD, MPH, FAAP
Chief, Division of Adolescent and Young Adult Medicine
Associate Professor
George Washington University School of Medicine and Health Sciences
Children's National Hospital
Washington, DC

Valerie N. Adams-Bass, PhD
Assistant Professor
Childhood Studies
Rutgers University
Camden, NJ

Hoover Adger Jr, MD, MPH, MBA, FAAP
Professor of Pediatrics
Division of Adolescent and Young Adult Medicine
Johns Hopkins University School of Medicine
Baltimore, MD

Nusheen Ameenuddin, MD, MPH, MPA, FAAP
Assistant Professor of Pediatrics
Mayo Clinic Children's Center
Mayo Clinic
Rochester, MN

Riana Elyse Anderson, PhD, LCP
Fellow
Center for Advanced Study in the Behavioral Sciences
Stanford University
Stanford, CA

Lee Savio Beers, MD, FAAP
Professor of Pediatrics
Child Health Advocacy Institute
Children's National Hospital
Washington, DC

Nathaniel Beers, MD, MPA, FAAP
Executive Vice President, Community and Population Health
Children's National Hospital
Clinical Professor of Pediatrics
George Washington University
Washington, DC

Harolyn M. E. Belcher, MD, MHS, FAAP
Vice President and Chief Diversity Officer
Director, Office for Health, Equity, Inclusion, and Diversity
Kennedy Krieger Institute
Professor of Pediatrics
Johns Hopkins University School of Medicine
Adjunct Appointment, Department of Mental Health
Johns Hopkins Bloomberg School of Public Health
Baltimore, MD

Nia Imani Bodrick, MD, MPH, FAAP
Attending Physician
Children's National Hospital
Assistant Professor of Pediatrics
George Washington University School of Medicine and Health Sciences
Washington, DC

Carmel Bogle, MD, FAAP
Assistant Professor of Pediatrics
Division of Pediatric Cardiology
Johns Hopkins Children's Center
Baltimore, MD

Alfiee M. Breland-Noble, PhD, MHSc
CEO, the Dr. Alfiee Org
Founder, The AAKOMA Project
Arlington, VA

Daniela Brissett, MD
Adolescent Medicine Fellow Physician
Craig-Dalsimer Division of Adolescent Medicine
Children's Hospital of Philadelphia
Philadelphia, PA

Merrian J. Brooks, DO, MS, FAAP
Assistant Professor of Pediatrics
Craig-Dalsimer Division of Adolescent Medicine
University of Pennsylvania
Perelman School of Medicine
Lead Physician, Botswana-UPenn Partnership
Philadelphia, PA

Camille Broussard, MD, MPH, FAAP
Assistant Professor of Pediatrics
Division of Adolescent and Young Adult Medicine
Johns Hopkins University School of Medicine
Baltimore, MD

Joseph Burns, MD, FAAP
Clinical Postdoctoral Fellow
Pediatric Cardiology
Baylor College of Medicine/Texas Children's Hospital
Houston, TX

Bethany L. Carlos, MD, MPH, FAAP
Pediatrician
Children's National Hospital
Climate and Health Equity Fellow
The Medical Society Consortium on Climate and Health
Washington, DC

Alexandra M. S. Corley, MD, MPH, FAAP
Assistant Professor of Pediatrics
Attending Physician
Division of General and Community Pediatrics
Cincinnati Children's Hospital Medical Center
University of Cincinnati College of Medicine
Cincinnati, OH

Tamera Coyne-Beasley, MD, MPH, FSAHM, FAAP
Derrol Dawkins MD Endowed Chair in Adolescent Medicine
Professor of Pediatrics and Internal Medicine
Vice Chair, Pediatrics for Community Engagement
Children's of Alabama
Birmingham, AL

Desiree M. de la Torre, MPH, MBA
Director
Community Affairs and Population Health Improvement
Children's National Hospital
Washington, DC

Gabrina L. Dixon, MD, MEd, FAAP
Associate Professor of Pediatrics
Attending Physician
Division of Hospital Medicine
Children's National Hospital
Washington, DC

Danielle G. Dooley, MD, MPhil, FAAP
Medical Director, Community Affairs and Population Health
Child Health Advocacy Institute
Children's National Hospital
Associate Professor of Pediatrics
George Washington University School of Medicine and Health Sciences
Washington, DC

Jacqueline Dougé, MD, MPH, FAAP
Assistant Professor of Public Health
Department of Nursing
Hood College
Frederick, MD

Nadia Dowshen, MD, MSHP
Director, Adolescent HIV Services
Craig-Dalsimer Division of Adolescent Medicine
Faculty, PolicyLab
Medical Director, Gender and Sexuality Development Program
Children's Hospital of Philadelphia
Associate Professor
Department of Pediatrics
University of Pennsylvania Perelman School of Medicine
Philadelphia, PA

Allison Empey, MD, FAAP (Confederated Tribes of Grand Ronde)
Assistant Professor
Division of General Pediatrics
Vice Chair of Equity, Diversity, and Inclusion
Department of Pediatrics
Oregon Health & Science University
Portland, OR

Olanrewaju Falusi, MD, MEd, FAAP
Medical Director of Advocacy Education
Child Health Advocacy Institute
Associate Program Director
Pediatric Residency Program
Attending Physician
Children's Health Center at Columbia Heights
Assistant Professor of Pediatrics
George Washington University School of Medicine and Health Sciences
Children's National Hospital
Washington, DC

Sarah Gaither, PhD
Nicolas J. and Theresa M. Leonardy Associate Professor of Psychology
    and Neuroscience
Duke University
Durham, NC

Kenneth R. Ginsburg, MD, MS Ed, FAAP
Professor of Pediatrics
Division of Adolescent Medicine
Children's Hospital of Philadelphia
Philadelphia, PA

Margaret A. Hagerman, PhD
Associate Professor of Sociology
Mississippi State University
Mississippi State, MS

Rachel Hardeman, PhD, MPH
Associate Professor
Blue Cross Endowed Professor of Health and Racial Equity
University of Minnesota School of Public Health
Founding Director
Center for Antiracism Research for Health Equity
Minneapolis, MN

Asha Hassan, MPH
Graduate Research Assistant
Center for Antiracism Research for Health Equity
Division of Health Policy and Management
University of Minnesota School of Public Health
Minneapolis, MN

Nevin J. Heard, PhD
Director of Intercultural Relations
Lake Forest College
Lake Forest, IL

Nia Heard-Garris, MD, MBA, MSc, FAAP
Assistant Professor of Pediatrics
Ann & Robert H. Lurie Children's Hospital of Chicago
Northwestern University School of Medicine
Chicago, IL

Benjamin D. Hoffman, MD, CPST-I, FAAP
Professor of Pediatrics
Oregon Health & Science University
Portland, OR

Diane L. Hughes, PhD
Professor of Applied Psychology
New York University
New York, NY

Meghan Drayton Jackson, DO, MBOE
Assistant Professor, Department of Pediatrics
Indiana University School of Medicine
Medical Director, Hematology Program
Director, Hematology/Oncology/BMT Quality Control
Division of Pediatric Hematology/Oncology
Riley Hospital for Children
Indianapolis, IN

Monique Jindal, MD, MPH, FAAP
Assistant Professor of Clinical Medicine
Department of Academic Internal Medicine
University of Illinois Chicago
Chicago, IL

Tiffani J. Johnson, MD, MSc, FAAP
Associate Professor of Emergency Medicine
University of California, Davis
Sacramento, CA

Vanya Jones, PhD, MPH
Assistant Professor
Johns Hopkins Bloomberg School of Public Health
Department of Health, Behavior and Society
Baltimore, MD

Jonathan Kang, MS
Doctoral Student
Counseling Psychology Program
Indiana University Bloomington
Bloomington, IN

J'Mag Karbeah, PhD, MPH
Assistant Professor
Division of Health Policy and Management
School of Public Health
University of Minnesota, Twin Cities
Minneapolis, MN

Julia M. Kim, MD, MPH, FAAP
Associate Vice Chair
Pediatric Ambulatory Quality and Safety
Johns Hopkins University School of Medicine
Baltimore, MD

Tonya Vidal Kinlow, MPA
Vice President, Community Engagement, Advocacy and
    Government Affairs
Children's National Hospital
Washington, DC

Joy A. Lewis, MSW, MPH
Senior Vice President
American Hospital Association
Washington, DC

Julie M. Linton, MD, FAAP
Associate Dean for Admissions
Associate Professor of Pediatrics
University of South Carolina School of Medicine Greenville
Prisma Health Upstate Children's Hospital
Greenville, SC

Gerri Mattson, MD, MSPH, FAAP
Adjunct Associate Professor
Department of Maternal and Child Health
Gillings School of Global Public Health
University of North Carolina
Chapel Hill, NC

Shruti Mittal, MD, FAAP
Assistant Professor
Developmental-Behavioral Pediatrics
Atrium Health Levine Children's Hospital
Charlotte, NC

Kristin Mmari, DrPH, MA
Associate Professor of American Health
Department of Population, Family, and Reproductive Health
Johns Hopkins Bloomberg School of Public Health
Baltimore, MD

Diana Montoya-Williams, MD, MSHP, FAAP
Assistant Professor of Pediatrics
Division of Neonatology
University of Pennsylvania Perelman School of Medicine
Children's Hospital of Philadelphia
Philadelphia, PA

Dipesh Navsaria, MD, MPH, MSLIS, FAAP
Professor (CHS) of Pediatrics
University of Wisconsin School of Medicine & Public Health
Clinical Professor of Human Development & Family Studies
School of Human Ecology, University of Wisconsin–Madison
Madison, WI

Rhodora Osborn, JD, LLM
Director, Organizational Equity
Johns Hopkins Health System
Baltimore, MD

Mikah Owen, MD, MPH, MBA, FAAP
Senior Clinical and Academic Program Director, Health Equity
UCLA-UCSF ACEs Aware Family Resilience Network
Sacramento, CA

Akilah Patterson, MPH
Doctoral Student
University of Michigan
School of Public Health
Ann Arbor, MI

Jerome A. Paulson, MD, FAAP
Professor Emeritus of Pediatrics and of Environmental & Occupational Health
George Washington University School of Medicine and Health Sciences
George Washington Milken Institute School of Public Health
Alexandria, VA

Silvia Pereira-Smith, MD, FAAP
Assistant Professor
Division of Developmental-Behavioral Pediatrics
Medical University of South Carolina
Charleston, SC

Marie Plaisime, PhD, MPH
Health and Human Rights Fellow
Harvard T. H. Chan School of Public Health
Boston, MA

Jean L. Raphael, MD, MPH, FAAP
Professor of Pediatrics
Division of Academic General Pediatrics
Baylor College of Medicine
Houston, TX

Renata Arrington Sanders, MD, MPH, ScM
Associate Professor of Pediatrics
Medical Director, Pediatric and Adolescent HIV/AIDS Program
Director of Pediatrics and Adolescent Services
Center for Transgender and Gender Expansive Health
Division of Adolescent and Young Adult Medicine
Baltimore, MD

Rahul Shah, MD, MBA, FAAP
Senior Vice President, Hospital-Based Specialties
Professor of Surgery and Pediatrics
George Washington University School of Medicine and Health Sciences
Washington, DC

Joshua M. Sharfstein, MD, FAAP
Professor of the Practice in Health Policy and Management
Johns Hopkins Bloomberg School of Public Health
Baltimore, MD

Michelle Spencer, MS
Associate Director, Bloomberg American Health Initiative
Associate Scientist, Department of Health Policy and Management
Associate Chair for Inclusion, Diversity, Anti-Racism, and Equity
Johns Hopkins Bloomberg School of Public Health
Baltimore, MD

Adiaha Spinks-Franklin, MD, MPH, FAAP
Clinical Associate Professor of Pediatrics
Baylor College of Medicine
Houston, TX

Brenda Straka, PhD
Assistant Professor
Department of Psychology
University of Illinois at Urbana-Champaign
Champaign, IL

María Verónica Svetaz, MD, MPH, FSAHM, FAAP
Associate Professor, Family and Community Medicine
University of Minnesota
Faculty, Medical Director
Hennepin Healthcare
Minneapolis, MN

Rachel L. J. Thornton, MD, PhD, FAAP
Vice President, Chief Health Equity Officer
Nemours Children's Health
Wilmington, DE

Maria Trent, MD, MPH, FSAHM, FAAP
Bloomberg Professor of American Health, Pediatrics, and Nursing
Senior Associate Dean of Diversity and Inclusive Excellence
Director, Division of Adolescent and Young Adult Medicine
Johns Hopkins University
Baltimore, MD

Megan R. Underhill, PhD
Associate Professor
Department of Sociology and Anthropology
University of North Carolina at Asheville
Asheville, NC

Stephenie Wallace, MD, MSPH, FAAP
Professor of Pediatrics
Division of Adolescent Medicine
University of Alabama at Birmingham
Birmingham, AL

Janie Victoria Ward, EdD
Professor Emerita
Department of Education and Africana Studies
Simmons University
Boston, MA

Bridget E. Weller, PhD
Professor of Social Work
Director of Research
College of Health and Human Services
Western Michigan University
Kalamazoo, MI

J. Deanna Wilson, MD, MPH
Presidential Assistant Professor
Department of Family Medicine and Community Health
University of Pennsylvania Perelman School of Medicine
Philadelphia, PA

Y. Joel Wong, PhD
Professor, Counseling Psychology Program
Indiana University Bloomington
Bloomington, IN

Joannie Yeh, MD, FAAP
Clinical Assistant Professor of Pediatrics
Media, PA

Equity, Diversity, and Inclusion Statement

The American Academy of Pediatrics is committed to principles of equity, diversity, and inclusion in its publishing program. Editorial boards, author selections, and author transitions (publication succession plans) are designed to include diverse voices that reflect society as a whole. Editor and author teams are encouraged to actively seek out diverse authors and reviewers at all stages of the editorial process. Publishing staff are committed to promoting equity, diversity, and inclusion in all aspects of publication writing, review, and production.

Contents

A Word From Our CEO/Executive Vice President

With this book, *Untangling the Thread of Racism: A Primer for Pediatric Health Professionals*, Maria Trent, MD, MPH; Danielle G. Dooley, MD, MPhil; and Jackie Dougé, MD, MPH, have made an important contribution to the role of medicine in overcoming the entrenched effects of racism in the lives and health of youth (children and adolescents). Although racial health disparities have been thoroughly cataloged, the social strategies, clinical interventions, and systemic reforms necessary to address them have lagged. Pediatricians and others who care for minoritized youth bear witness in frustration while demanding urgent change. For many, this happens as they confront racism in their professional settings and lives.

Pediatricians have always considered factors outside the examination room that affect the lives of their patients. Long before there was a term for social determinants of health, pediatricians understood that much of what influences the health of their patients happens in families, communities, and the environments in which they live, work, and play. From the earliest days of the American Academy of Pediatrics (AAP), its mission has focused on caring for youth's physical health and improving their lives and well-being. The first president of the AAP, Isaac Abt, MD, said in his 1931 presidential address, "As an organization, we should assist and lead in public health measures, social reform, and hospital and educational administration as they affect the welfare of children." In 2019, the AAP policy statement "The Impact of Racism on Child and Adolescent Health" identified racism as a core social determinant of health. With that statement, confronting and dismantling systemic racism became rooted in the mission of the AAP, finally locating anti-racism in the "social reform" the founders envisioned. In 2020, we engaged in a truth and reconciliation process that moved us beyond what should occur in clinical practice and as professionals, leaders, and an organization. We acknowledged past discrimination in the history of the AAP. We held a referendum resulting in the broad adoption of nondiscrimination policies as we work together for youth and families.

Today, AAP efforts to achieve equity, diversity, and inclusion for all youth must be guided by scholarship and real-world implementation tools. This book offers a road map for pediatric health professionals to understand how racism impedes optimal pediatric practice, challenges the healthy development of youth, undermines communities, and weakens our nation. It then guides readers to strategies and solutions for clinical settings, health systems, public health, and public policy.

For too many patients, this book is urgently needed. For racism, like other social determinants of health, change begins in the powerful personal interactions between patients and their clinicians and among colleagues. Still, it must extend to clinical guidance, health institutions, biomedical research, and communities to fully integrate with public health and optimize outcomes.

Systemic problems require systemic solutions. As the authors of Section 3, Public Health, Policy, and Advocacy, teach us, public policy change through organized and sustained advocacy is needed. Policy makers have perhaps the most essential role in unwinding the laws, government institutions, and administrative rules that have enabled and reinforced racial inequity and their associated health outcomes and disparities. For pediatric health professionals and all who care for children, this book is a reminder of the unique responsibility to advocate for change while providing the best care. Thankfully, this book can help with both.

Mark Del Monte, JD
CEO/Executive Vice President
American Academy of Pediatrics

Foreword

As a prelude to the publication of this primer, over the past 5 years, the American Academy of Pediatrics (AAP) has amplified and contributed significantly to the evidentiary basis for addressing racism. Beginning with the landmark 2019 policy statement, "The Impact of Racism on Child and Adolescent Health," which was the first such statement to call racism by its name and establish addressing it as an organizational priority, the AAP has steadfastly continued, in the words of Janie Victoria Ward, EdD, a contributor to this primer, "to recognize racism in all its forms, call it explicitly by name, declaratively oppose it, and exercise commitment and resolve to actively replace it." The AAP has built on the recommendations of "The Impact of Racism on Child and Adolescent Health," also authored by this primer's editors, Maria Trent, MD, MPH; Danielle G. Dooley, MD, MPhil; and Jackie Dougé, MD, MPH, to establish further policy on dismantling race-based approaches to the delivery of clinical care and to the creation of AAP educational content. The AAP and its governance have also established a detailed health equity work plan to define the path to anti-racism within pediatrics. With this framework in mind, the contributors to *Untangling the Thread of Racism: A Primer for Pediatric Health Professionals* bring synergistic scholarship to the subject of racism and its effects on children, adolescents, and families.

Notably, the editors have organized the primer's content such that the chapters can be actively used as discrete, fund-of-knowledge–enhancing modules or continuously absorbed as an unprecedented, authoritative subject-matter–expertise collection to be repeatedly referenced like an encyclopedia. This aspect of the content presentation is essential because, as readers, we are all at different places on our anti-racism journeys and bring unique differential knowledge and lived experiences to the table. Having available an evidence-informed resource such as *Untangling the Thread of Racism: A Primer for Pediatric Health Professionals* allows us to learn incrementally and build awareness and knowledge longitudinally— similarly to the way that children are socialized to the role of race and racism in our society across critical stages in their development. Incorporating the principles of racial socialization, spanning an array of settings and involving diverse populations, is an indispensable feature that foundationally undergirds the primer's parts and sections. Intersectionality, one of the gap analysis content areas identified by the AAP Task Force on Addressing Bias and Discrimination, is undertaken by the primer in several chapters.

Moving forward, and not dissimilar from the catalyst that "The Impact of Racism on Child and Adolescent Health" has broadly provided for the field of equity and health equity, I fully expect *Untangling the Thread of Racism: A Primer for Pediatric Health Professionals* to be a bibliometric accelerant to the academic literature in this area that will contribute to a reframing of the science of health equity through an anti-racist lens. Debunking unsubstantiated science and challenging perpetu-ated myths with contemporary objectivity and viewpoints is critical to progress along the anti-racism journey. There is no question that the moral imperative to tackle racism is primary and paramount and must be top of mind for all pediat-ric health professionals. Yet we must equivalently apply due diligence, rigor, and thought leadership to this work's evidence generation and subsequent dissemi-nation. *Untangling the Thread of Racism: A Primer for Pediatric Health Professionals* authentically and unequivocally rises to the task.

Joseph L. Wright, MD, MPH

Chief Health Equity Officer/SVP, Equity Initiatives

American Academy of Pediatrics

Acknowledgments

To my mom, Vivian Trent, who prepared me to face the constantly contemporary nature of racism and the positive impacts of making "good trouble." To my husband, Dr Gregory Hampton, who encouraged me to unapologetically leverage critical inquiry to write about what others often can't or don't want to see. To my children, Safi and Hodari, who have brought so much light into my life and inspire me to keep moving, as they are a daily reminder of what's at stake. And finally, thank you to Danielle, Jackie, and our collaborators who fearlessly stand with me on the forefront of change. —MT

To John, exemplary husband, father, and physician, who makes all things possible for our family and who is my greatest champion. To Catherine and Jack, you are my everything and the reason I do what I do. Watching you navigate the world with kindness, humor, compassion, and joy inspires me every day. To my parents, Collette and Allan, for their examples of public service. To my brothers, George and AJ, the best people to grow up with and go through life with. To Vanessa, who makes it possible for me to go to work each day. To my in-laws, Abby, Melanie, Tony, Noël, Chris, Ann Marie, Drew, Daniel, and Alison, thank you for supporting me in so many ways—and for the fun! To all the patients and families I have been honored to care for, thank you for showing me how to be a better pediatrician and parent. To Maria and Jackie, we have navigated the highest highs and the lowest lows together in life, and I admire you both beyond measure. —DGD

I would like to express my heartfelt gratitude to my husband, Max, and our 2 sons, Malcolm and Emmanuel. Your unwavering support and love have been my constant inspiration. Additionally, I would like to extend my appreciation to my dear friends and coeditors, Danielle Dooley and Maria Trent. Working with such remarkable women has been an incredible experience. —JD

Introduction

In the summer of 2019, after a series of tragedies across the United States emerging from racism and other forms of discrimination, the American Academy of Pediatrics quietly published a policy statement entitled "The Impact of Racism on Child and Adolescent Health." While almost 2 years in the making, from conception to publication, it facilitated a shift in the work of the world's oldest and largest pediatric organization—internally and externally. Internally, the organization completed a truth and reconciliation process with a referendum on an antidiscrimination policy and launched a strategic plan with diversity, inclusion, and health equity at its core. Externally, events such as the deadly El Paso shooting targeted the Latinx community and took the lives of adults and 3 children aged 2, 9, and 15 years almost simultaneously with the statement's release. The queries our leaders received pushed this advocacy organization of pediatricians further into the health equity work as our now intersecting organizational policies against both gun violence and discrimination were clear.

Pediatric health professionals have committed their life's work to the care and well-being of infants, children, adolescents, and families. Yet we learned from the truth and reconciliation process that we are all products of our social, developmental, and environmental contexts. Essentially, these experiences have shaped the lens through which we view the world as adults and influence our conscious and unconscious behaviors as we navigate daily life. The world has also been changing, with infants, children, adolescents, and families—and the pediatric health professionals who serve them—facing new challenges. Many of these challenges relate to the forces that question the value of understanding history to prevent reoccurring traumas that seep into the psyche and inflict harm that shapes the potential outcomes for young people. For example, although race is well established as a social construct, the trauma of racism has persisted over generations, resulting in differential health and social well-being outcomes that are difficult to escape. Even terms once considered progressive, such as *woke*, a term meant to describe those enlightened to social justice issues, have become a moniker of something detrimental to society, undermining the environments in which children grow, live, learn, and play. We must understand that our role is to ensure that adults, including us, are not asleep, impaired, or oblivious at the wheel but are truly alert and empowered to drive child health and development. We must use our training and gifts to educate and provide patient-centered, family-engaged care and support to ensure that every child meets their optimal developmental outcomes and personal goals. This commitment also means we need space to reflect, learn, and equip ourselves with knowledge, strategies, and tools to implement best practices and policies.

This work also embraces the ambiguity of the evolving language of diversity, equity, and inclusion while acknowledging the challenges of identities being shaped by our increasingly heterogeneous society. Throughout the text, there will be some variability by the author in describing where the intersectionality of self- or community-described race and ethnicity versus socially structured identities collides. For example, *Black* represents a government-defined racial construct and, later, an empowerment strategy for embracing *Blackness*, while *African American* represents bridging African ancestry with an American identity. These terms may still not include individuals with similar origins who leverage a more refined specificity to African-based identities (eg, Afro-Caribbean, Afro-Latino, African). Use of the term *Hispanic* is contemporary, with first use implemented in the 1980s by the US government in data collection procedures to reference the Spanish-speaking populations who advocated for a category that would afford them deserved opportunities. As a result, *Latino* emerged as a more prevailing self-defining and empowering term, especially to disconnect Latin America from Spain and its role in colonialism. This book uses a combination of *Latine*, *Latine/x*, *Latino/a*, *Latino/a/e*, and *Latinx* as gender-neutral and/or gender-inclusive alternatives to *Latino*, recognizing that the terms have been continually evolving and many Latinx people and groups may use specific countries of origin (eg, Brazilian, Cuban, Puerto Rican) to describe themselves and their communities. The aforementioned terms and others such as *Asian American/Pacific Islander* and *American Indian/Alaska Native* present an aggregate view of individuals. In these ambiguous spaces, we meet patients and families humbly and earnestly to learn their perspectives and preferences while embracing intersectionality (eg, country of origin, immigration status, gender, sexuality, ability) that may influence health status. Finally, we recognize that white children, adolescents, and families are not a monolith and that racism affects them in ways that few people have studied, so we devote time to considering how to create healthy strategies that enable them to navigate race and racism as well.

Based on the publication data from the policy statement, there has been tremendous interest in the policy statement, leaving clinicians and other pediatric health professionals asking about the how-to of executing the policy recommendations and addressing racism more broadly. Our shared goal is to provide pediatric health professionals with materials they can easily access and use to engage in transformative change within clinical, administrative, research, public health, and policy settings. We also remain aligned with the American Academy of Pediatrics policy statement goals to advance the strategic agenda to eliminate racism as a cause of infant, child, and adolescent health disparities. We envisioned this primer as the next step in providing the opportunity for pediatric health professionals to deepen their understanding of racism and of how to minimize unconscious and perhaps conscious biases within themselves, their clinical practices, and their more expansive roles as leaders within their institutions and the local community. For this work, we have harnessed perspectives and voices intimately engaged in work that explores the social frameworks through which racism exerts itself on infants, children, adolescents, families, communities, institutions, and structures that, in turn, shape the health, developmental, educational, legal, and economic outcomes for those we serve. Although not exhaustive, we hope that it is sufficiently expansive and accessible for considering key issues to improve one's relational reality with race and racism and that it optimizes interpersonal communication, professionalism, advocacy, and leadership. As such, this book, designed for the busy professional, is divided into 3 moments: the first focuses on framing issues; the second, on understanding the intersections of race and health for infants, children, and adolescents, with some focus on population-specific issues and community experiences of racism; and the third, on optimizing anti-racism in practice. Ultimately, we hope the reader will improve their practice and beyond by challenging and changing practice and policies and disrupting business as usual in medicine to achieve racial justice and optimize health outcomes across the infant, child, adolescent, and emerging adult life course.

The best part of this collaborative work is that we have continued to build on our existing relationship and are bonded through our shared interests, research, and writing. We have also shared meals and personal details of our lives and created new or strengthened relationships with the many authors who have graciously contributed to this project. We have found that as an editorial team, we are professional women, scientists, public health professionals, advocates, and mothers. We are more similar than different, with intersecting timelines, identities, and life experiences. We have experienced grief, angst, change, challenges, and tremendous joy as we have navigated the policy statement and this book project together. Most importantly, we have again dipped our toes into this space to become more powerful advocates for infants, children, adolescents, and families in collaboration with patients, families, communities, and institutions. We hope you will take the next step with us to proactively untangle the threads of racism woven into our history that stagnate our present so we can create a better world for the next generation.

Part 1. Framing the Issues

CHAPTER 1

Moving Toward Health Equity

Jacqueline Dougé, MD, MPH, and Gerri Mattson, MD, MSPH

The idea that some lives matter less is the root of all that is wrong with the world.

Paul Farmer, MD, PhD

Introduction

The United States has not attained health equity, or the "highest level of health for all people."[1] Communities that have been racially marginalized continue to face barriers to fair and just opportunities and therefore experience poorer health outcomes. As a recent example, during the COVID-19 pandemic, Black, Latinx[a], and Native American/Alaska Native populations experienced higher rates of infection, more serious cases of illness, and higher rates of death from COVID-19.[2,3] However, these health inequities, or "systemic differences in the health status of different population groups,"[4] are caused not by race or ethnicity but by the systemic racism that belies their identities. For this chapter, we leverage the definition of racism as "a system of structuring opportunity and assigning value based on the social interpretation of how one looks that unfairly disadvantages some individuals and communities, unfairly advantages other individuals and communities, and saps the strength of the whole society through the waste of human resources."[5] This chapter discusses how structural racism affects health equity and how the discussion of collaboration with diverse partners, data, advocacy, and screening for social determinants of health (SDOH) can improve the health of all children.

Health Equity and Structural Racism

Despite historical progress in the advancement of civil rights, racism continues to negatively affect the ability of all children and families to experience health equity, or have opportunities to achieve their full health potential.[6-9] Racism impedes access to quality health care, housing, education and employment, and fair treatment in the criminal justice system for populations that have been racially minoritized, subsequently referred to as *minoritized populations.*[6-8]

Structural racism is a term that can further describe a type of racism that is "pervasively and deeply embedded in systems, laws, written or unwritten policies, and entrenched practices and beliefs that produce, condone, and perpetuate widespread unfair treatment

---

[a] In this chapter, we use Latinx when referring to people of Latin American origin or descent as a whole. It is a gender-neutral and gender-inclusive alternative to Latino. For a brief history of this term, including a rationale, refer to the book introduction.

and oppression of people of color, with adverse health consequences."[10] Structural racism creates discriminatory and prejudicial policies and processes within neighborhoods, businesses, institutions, and systems.[10] These unjust policies and processes have resulted in many Black, Hispanic, and American Indian/Alaska Native individuals and communities experiencing air and water pollution, unfair policing, and the discriminatory practice of loan refusals or redlining, which is associated with poor health and well-being.[6–8,11]

Pediatric health professionals have evolved in our understanding of health inequities, and we are working to move beyond the practice of identifying health disparities, or "differences in health and well-being outcomes without an identified cause among groups of people."[2] The goal has become to identify the causes of these differences and to work toward a state of health equity, in which "everyone has the opportunity to attain full health potential and no one is disadvantaged from achieving this potential because of social position or any other socially defined circumstance."[9] Efforts toward achieving health equity now include recognizing and addressing the role that racism plays in creating disadvantages in access to opportunities (ie, jobs, housing, health care) and, therefore, differences in health and well-being.

The term *health disparities* defines only the differences in health outcomes. Historically, health disparities have been associated with racial differences, instead of racism, as an important SDOH. Structural racism has been embedded within policies, laws, practices, and institutions that have created poorer health outcomes for children and adolescents in minoritized populations. There are several key areas that pediatric health professionals and teams can address to achieve health equity. These areas include advocating for more inclusive data on race and ethnicity, collaborating with diverse key partners, advocating for more research on health equity and its impact on minoritized populations, and screening for and addressing SDOH. The journey toward health equity for children is better when all systems of care agree that health equity is a priority and an achievable goal.

Pursuing Health Equity for Children

The journey toward health equity begins with attention to key areas to determine how racism may be operating to create health inequities.[12,13] Fundamental steps follow.

Screening for and Addressing Social Determinants of Health

Pediatric health professionals and teams can play an important role in screening for and addressing SDOH during clinical encounters. Chapter 2, Social Determinants of Health and the Invisible Ubiquity of Racism: A Driving Force of Health Inequities and the Way Forward, further describes their effects and how racism is considered an SDOH.

Data

Pediatric health professionals and researchers can ask for and use data that are inclusive of race and ethnicity to understand a baseline and what is being measured and to serve as a barometer of improvement in health outcomes across all populations (refer to Chapter 32, Pediatric and Adolescent Research on Race and Racism, for a more detailed discussion).

Advocacy

Pediatric health professionals can advocate for expanded funding for research on health equity and its impact on minoritized populations and can implement the principles and policies of health equity into practice, policy development, and research (refer to Chapter 33, Child Health Advocacy and Anti-racism, for a more detailed discussion).

Collaborating With Diverse Key Partners

Pediatric health professionals can collaborate with and strengthen relationships with diverse key partners in the community that have shared goals and interactions related to the health and well-being of children. Examples of partners include community-based organizations, nonprofit organizations, local health departments, and school systems.

American Academy of Pediatrics Equity Agenda

The American Academy of Pediatrics Equity Agenda has a set of key principles (Box 1–1) that can serve as touchstones to help guide pediatric health professionals and teams toward promoting and achieving health equity in partnership with others.[14]

Box 1–1.

Principles From the American Academy of Pediatrics Equity Agenda

1. All children and adolescents have equitable health care within a medical home that includes primary care, subspecialty services, emergency medical services, and hospital care.
2. Child and adolescent health care professionals shall address the social, behavioral, and environmental factors that affect children's health, development, and achievement.
3. Child and adolescent health care professionals deliver care in a culturally and linguistically effective manner that addresses the unique needs of each child and family.
4. Child and adolescent health care professionals deliver care based on the best available evidence.
5. Child and adolescent health care professionals advocate for identification and elimination of racist policies and the inequities that contribute to racial disparities and impede equity.
6. Child and adolescent health care is delivered using language that the patient and family prefer.
7. Child and adolescent health care delivery settings are welcoming and reflect the diversity of their patients.
8. Child and adolescent health care professionals receive training on delivering culturally and linguistically effective care.
9. The child and adolescent health care workforce is diverse and reflective of the child population.
10. Child and adolescent health care services are evaluated using data stratified by insurance status, race and ethnicity, language, socioeconomic status, gender, gender identity, religion, disability, and sexual orientation.

Summary

It is the time for pediatric health professionals and teams to move beyond addressing health disparities and instead pursue health equity. Currently, much of the work we do is done in isolation, without the benefit of working with other professionals in the community who have shared goals and interactions with our patients and families. The goal of eliminating health inequities and achieving health equity must be integrated across systems of care, such as those of health, education, economy, and government, for all children and families to thrive.

References

1. Office of Disease Prevention and Health Promotion, US Department of Health and Human Services. Health Equity in Healthy People 2030. Healthy People 2030. Accessed March 13, 2023. https://health.gov/healthypeople/priority-areas/health-equity-healthy-people-2030

2. Gómez CA, Kleinman DV, Pronk N, et al. Addressing health equity and social determinants of health through Healthy People 2030. *J Public Health Manag Pract*. 2021;27(suppl 6):S249–S257 doi: 10.1097/PHH.0000000000001297

3. Office of Minority Health, US Department of Health and Human Services. Health disparities. Native American Heritage Month. Accessed July 22, 2023. https://minorityhealth.hhs.gov/nahm/health-disparities

4. World Health Organization. Health inequities and their causes. Published February 22, 2018. Accessed January 24, 2023. https://www.who.int/news-room/facts-in-pictures/detail/health-inequities-and-their-causes

5. Jones CP, Truman BI, Elam-Evans LD, et al. Using "socially assigned race" to probe white advantages in health status. *Ethn Dis*. 2008;18(4):496–504 PMID: 19157256

6. Bhopal R. Spectre of racism in health and health care: lessons from history and the United States. *BMJ*. 1998;316(7149):1970–1973 doi: 10.1136/bmj.316.7149.1970

7. Hahn RA, Truman BI, Williams DR. Civil rights as determinants of public health and racial and ethnic health equity: health care, education, employment, and housing in the United States. *SSM Popul Health*. 2018;4:17–24

8. Bailey ZD, Krieger N, Agénor M, Graves J, Linos N, Bassett MT. Structural racism and health inequities in the USA: evidence and interventions. *Lancet*. 2017;389(10077):1453–1463

9. Committee on Community-Based Solutions to Promote Health Equity in the United States, Board on Population Health and Public Health Practice, Health and Medicine Division, National Academies of Sciences, Engineering, and Medicine. *Communities in Action: Pathways to Health Equity*. Weinstein JN, Geller A, Negussie Y, Baciu A, eds. National Academies Press; 2017

10. Braveman PA, Arkin E, Proctor D, Kauh T, Holm N. Systemic and structural racism: definitions, examples, health damages, and approaches to dismantling. *Health Aff (Millwood)*. 2022;41(2):171–178. Accessed January 24, 2023. https://www.healthaffairs.org/doi/10.1377/hlthaff.2021.01394

11. Pager D, Shepherd H. The sociology of discrimination: racial discrimination in employment, housing, credit, and consumer markets. *Annu Rev Sociol.* 2008;34:181–209. Accessed January 24, 2023. https://www.ncbi.nlm.nih.gov/pmc/articles/PMC2915460

12. Trent M, Dooley DG, Dougé J; American Academy of Pediatrics Section on Adolescent Health, Council on Community Pediatrics, and Committee on Adolescence. The impact of racism on child and adolescent health. *Pediatrics.* 2019;144(2):e20191765

13. Montoya-Williams D, Peña MM, Fuentes-Afflick E. In pursuit of health equity in pediatrics. *J Pediatr X.* 2020;5:100045 doi: 10.1016/j.ympdx.2020.100045

14. American Academy of Pediatrics. AAP Equity Agenda. Accessed January 24, 2023. https://www.aap.org/en/about-the-aap/american-academy-of-pediatrics-equity-and-inclusion-efforts/aap-equity-agenda

Social Determinants of Health and the Invisible Ubiquity of Racism: A Driving Force of Health Inequities and the Way Forward

Rachel L. J. Thornton, MD, PhD

Introduction

Childhood is a time when people are generally healthy. Yet children's and adolescents' negative experiences, exposures, and environments as they grow can produce illness, injury, trauma, or even chronic disease that manifests later in life.[1,2] Often referred to as the *social determinants of health* (SDOH),[3] the political, economic, social, and environmental conditions in which children grow, learn, live, and play can lead to lifelong impacts on health and well-being.

The SDOH are fundamental drivers of health disparities in the United States. Sentinel work by W. E. B. DuBois[4-6] laid bare the role of racism in creating and maintaining the economic and political conditions in the United States that produce and sustain disparities. This work made it clear that poverty, education, employment, housing, and neighborhood conditions do not exist in isolation; rather, they are organized in ways that work together to produce disproportionately adverse health effects for groups at the bottom of the racial hierarchy.

Pediatric clinical and population health efforts are increasingly focused on the SDOH, with particular attention placed on individual social needs affecting patients or families.[7,8] It is critical for pediatric health professionals to identify and address unmet needs (eg, housing, poverty, and food insecurity) with patients and families during clinical encounters to help connect them to available resources in the community. However, although this approach helps individual families, it does not produce a positive change in community conditions.[8] For example, screening a patient for food insecurity in a clinic provides an opportunity to address their immediate needs, but screening and connecting individuals to services does not address the shared root causes of unmet needs that result from the SDOH in communities (eg, concentrated poverty, inadequate affordable housing supply, or lack of access to employment, high-quality educational opportunities, transportation, or healthful and affordable food).

Identified: Housing

The intergenerational impacts of housing and neighborhood conditions on the health and well-being of children and families are substantial. For example, several studies, including primary and secondary analyses of data from the Moving to Opportunity for Fair Housing Demonstration trial, have examined the effect of moving from a high- to low-poverty neighborhood on health outcomes of caregivers and children with low or very low incomes.[2,9,10] These studies highlight the cumulative impacts on the development of a child and the physical and behavioral health outcomes associated with concentrated poverty.

Addressing: Housing

Although safe, stable, affordable housing is a prerequisite for health, there is a long-standing housing insecurity crisis in the United States. When families with children are living in poverty, it disproportionately places them at risk for housing instability. They face significant excess rent burden, elevated risk for eviction, and numerous barriers in access to stable and affordable housing in safe and economically thriving neighborhoods. As with poverty, children from groups that have been historically marginalized face a disproportionately elevated risk for housing insecurity, homelessness, and substandard living conditions in the United States.[11]

Regrettably, affordable housing is not an entitlement for those whose incomes meet the eligibility criteria. As a result, the population whose incomes meet the eligibility criteria far outstrips the affordable housing subsidies available. The history of access to affordable rental housing and home ownership is often highlighted as emblematic of the impact of systemic and structural racism and its effects on other SDOH.[6,12–15]

Identified: Poverty

In the United States, children live in poverty at higher rates than adults. In 2019, 10.4% of the US population lived in poverty, yet 14.4% of these people were children. Since the global COVID-19 pandemic, the proportion of the population living in poverty has increased and children have remained disproportionately overrepresented. Contrary to some popular perceptions that when children experiencing poverty are from certain racial and ethnic groups, they are living in households in which their parents do not work, most children in families with limited incomes have at least one parent in the household who is working full-time.[16] According to the Children's Defense Fund, 71% of children living in poverty are children of color, with approximately 1 in 4 Black children and 1 in 5 Latinx[a] and Native American children living in poverty compared with 1 in 12 white and 1 in 14 Asian American, Native Hawaiian, or Pacific Islander children.[12,17–19]

---

[a] In this chapter, we use *Latinx* when referring to people of Latin American origin or descent as a whole. It is a gender-neutral and gender-inclusive alternative to *Latino*. For a brief history of this term, including a rationale, refer to the book introduction.

Not only are children of color more likely to live in households experiencing poverty, Black and Latinx children nationally live in neighborhoods with much less opportunity (as measured by the Child Opportunity Index) than white children, thus increasing their risk of living in neighborhoods that undermine optimal health.[20] Further, child poverty rates have exceeded 40% among Native American/Alaska Native children for the past 3 decades.[21]

Addressing: Poverty

The National Academies of Sciences, Engineering, and Medicine *A Roadmap to Reducing Child Poverty*[7] highlights the importance of so-called safety net programs and the expansion of economic supports tied to work in reducing child poverty. These strategies include means-tested and universal programs to increase income (eg, Earned Income Tax Credit program, Child Tax Credit program, work incentive programs, and raising of the minimum wage) and to reduce the economic burdens on families through subsidies (eg, nutrition assistance, housing assistance, child care assistance).

Identified: Food Insecurity

In 2019, approximately 20 million children in the United States received Supplemental Nutrition Assistance Program (SNAP) benefits, a statistic highlighting the significant effect of this program on the nutritional status of families and children living in poverty. In 2016, approximately 30% of SNAP funding went to Black participants. On average, Black households, which experience the highest rates of poverty in the United States, had an income at 56% of the federal poverty threshold, with a considerable proportion living in deep poverty. Similarly, the Latinx US population experiences higher rates of poverty than the overall US population, with 25% of SNAP funding going to Latinx families with an average monthly income at 59% of the federal poverty threshold.[22-24]

Addressing: Food Insecurity

Along with SNAP, the Special Supplemental Nutrition Assistance Program for Women, Infants, and Children and the US Department of Agriculture School Breakfast Program and National School Lunch Program provide children from families with limited incomes with optimal nutrition. A variety of factors may affect enrollment and participation in benefit programs, including what has been referred to as the "chilling effect" among immigrant families or among mixed-status households (eg, children who are US citizens and others who are not and who are likely ineligible for public assistance). For example, recent federal regulatory changes to the public charge rule have raised concern about immigrant families who have children with US citizenship yet forego public benefits for fear that it will expose them to immigration enforcement or other scrutiny. Although research analyzing impacts of the chilling effect are not conclusive, it is also possible that the chilling effect may extend to other public benefits programs (eg, Supplemental Security Income and Medicaid).[25-29]

Racism as a Social Determinant of Health

Despite widespread recognition of the effect that SDOH have on child and adolescent health trajectories, many efforts to address them through screening and interventions either ignore racism as a fundamental driver or erroneously conflate race and poverty. The American Academy of Pediatrics policy statement on poverty[30] acknowledges the disproportionate exposure to poverty and related SDOH for children from groups that have been historically marginalized. Still, it fails to situate child poverty within the context of racism as a structural force and SDOH. This attitude has impeded understanding and acceptance of racism itself as an SDOH.[5,6,31,32]

Pediatric health professionals and researchers must develop a more nuanced understanding of racism as an SDOH. The American Academy of Pediatrics policy statement describing the impact of racism on child health[33] lays a solid foundation for pediatric health professionals to build on. According to the policy statement, professionals in the field of pediatrics need to understand and explicitly call out the role of racism as an SDOH in US society and the interconnectedness of racial stratification as a contributor and perpetrator of inequities in child health that intersects with other contextual sources of disadvantage and adversity. That means identifying and addressing racism as a threat to child health and developing interventions that explicitly address this threat.

A Path Forward: Examples of Addressing Social Determinants of Health

Pediatric health professionals have opportunities to address the SDOH. They should screen for unmet social needs, refer patients to available resources, and maintain clear records to assess and understand the patterns of unmet social needs among their patient populations. Pediatric health professionals should work with analytic teams, public health departments, and others to characterize the sociodemographic and geographic patterns of unmet social needs across their patient populations, overlaying these patterns with a clear understanding of shared community exposures and conditions to inform advocacy efforts. Once they are equipped with this information, they must raise their voices and partner with providers and advocates in social services and other sectors, including economic development, employment, housing, community development, and education, to advocate for expanded investments that bolster access to goods, services, and environments that support healthy growth and development. That means refocusing some efforts from a solitary focus on treating illness once it emerges to an expanded focus on ensuring investments that bolster healthy trajectories and reduce the risk for illness in childhood.

Summary

For pediatric health professionals seeking to advance child health equity, understanding disparate social conditions within the context of racism as a structural force is critical. Equipped with this knowledge, we can continue efforts to address urgent unmet social needs among our patients. Simultaneously, we can examine how health care delivery, medical education, access to economic opportunity, and essential goods and services are distributed in our local communities, states, and nation. When our screenings and referrals reveal patterns of disadvantage or disinvestment, we must band together to raise the alarm and advocate for community investment in social services, economic development, education, and affordable housing resources—because we can amplify the voices of children and families that would otherwise go unheard.

References

1. National Research Council, Institute of Medicine. *From Neurons to Neighborhoods: The Science of Early Childhood Development.* Shonkoff JP, Phillips DA, eds. National Academies Press; 2000 doi: 10.17226/9824
2. Committee on Applying Neurobiological and Socio-behavioral Sciences From Prenatal Through Early Childhood Development: A Health Equity Approach, Board on Population Health and Public Health Practice, Health and Medicine Division, National Academies of Sciences, Engineering, and Medicine. *Vibrant and Healthy Kids: Aligning Science, Practice, and Policy to Advance Health Equity.* DeVoe JE, Geller A, Negussie Y, eds. National Academies Press; 2019 doi: 10.17226/25466
3. World Health Organization. Social determinants of health. Accessed January 25, 2023. https://www.who.int/health-topics/social-determinants-of-health
4. DuBois WEB. *The Philadelphia Negro: A Social Study.* University of Pennsylvania Press; 1899
5. White A, Thornton RLJ, Greene JA. Remembering past lessons about structural racism—recentering Black theorists of health and society. *N Engl J Med.* 2021;385(9):850–855 PMID: 34469642 doi: 10.1056/NEJMms2035550
6. Zambrana RE, Williams DR. The intellectual roots of current knowledge on racism and health: relevance to policy and the national equity discourse. *Health Aff (Millwood).* 2022;41(2):163–170 PMID: 35130075 doi: 10.1377/hlthaff.2021.01439
7. National Academies of Sciences, Engineering, and Medicine Committee on Building an Agenda to Reduce the Number of Children in Poverty by Half in 10 Years. *A Roadmap to Reducing Child Poverty.* Duncan G, Le Menestrel S, eds. National Academies Press; 2019 doi: 10.17226/25246
8. Thornton RLJ, Yang TJ. Addressing population health inequities: investing in the social determinants of health for children and families to advance child health equity. *Curr Opin Pediatr.* 2023;35(1):8–13 PMID: 36301135 doi: 10.1097/MOP.0000000000001189
9. Ludwig J, Sanbonmatsu L, Gennetian L, et al. Neighborhoods, obesity, and diabetes—a randomized social experiment. *N Engl J Med.* 2011;365(16):1509–1519 PMID: 22010917 doi: 10.1056/NEJMsa1103216
10. Chetty R, Hendren N, Katz LF. The effects of exposure to better neighborhoods on children: new evidence from the moving to opportunity experiment. *Am Econ Rev.* 2016;106(4):855–902 PMID: 29546974 doi: 10.1257/aer.20150572
11. Biennial worst case housing needs assessment reveals ongoing challenges in years before pandemic. US Department of Housing and Urban Development. October 26, 2021. Accessed June 1, 2023. https://www.huduser.gov/portal/pdredge/pdr-edge-research-102621.html
12. National Academies of Sciences, Engineering, and Medicine. *Rental Eviction and the COVID-19 Pandemic: Averting a Looming Crisis.* National Academies Press; 2022 doi: 10.17226/26106
13. Bostic RW, Thornton RLJ, Rudd EC, Sternthal MJ. Health in all policies: the role of the US Department of Housing and Urban Development and present and future challenges. *Health Aff (Millwood).* 2012;31(9):2130–2137 PMID: 22914341 doi: 10.1377/hlthaff.2011.1014
14. Pietila A. *Not in My Neighborhood: How Bigotry Shaped a Great American City.* Ivan R. Dee; 2010
15. Thornton RLJ, Glover CM, Cené CW, Glik DC, Henderson JA, Williams DR. Evaluating strategies for reducing health disparities by addressing the social determinants of health. *Health Aff (Millwood).* 2016;35(8):1416–1423 PMID: 27503966 doi: 10.1377/hlthaff.2015.1357

16. Koball H, Jiang Y. Basic facts about low-income children under 18 years, 2016. Fact sheet. National Center for Children in Poverty. January 2018. Accessed May 22, 2023. http://www.nccp.org/wp-content/uploads/2018/01/text_1194.pdf

17. US Census Bureau. Income, poverty and health insurance coverage in the United States: 2020. Accessed January 25, 2023. https://www.census.gov/newsroom/press-releases/2021/income-poverty-health-insurance-coverage.html

18. Gorski PA, Kuo AA, Granado-Villar DC, et al; American Academy of Pediatrics Council on Community Pediatrics. Community pediatrics: navigating the intersection of medicine, public health, and social determinants of children's health. *Pediatrics*. 2013;131(3):623–628 doi: 10.1542/peds.2012-3933

19. Dawson B. The State of America's Children 2021: child poverty. Children's Defense Fund. Accessed January 25, 2023. https://www.childrensdefense.org/state-of-americas-children/soac-2021-child-poverty

20. Acevedo-Garcia D, Noelke C, McArdle N, et al. Racial and ethnic inequities in children's neighborhoods: evidence from the new Child Opportunity Index 2.0. *Health Aff (Millwood)*. 2020;39(10):1693–1701 PMID: 33017244 doi: 10.1377/hlthaff.2020.00735

21. Akee R. How does measuring poverty and welfare affect American Indian children? Brookings. March 12, 2019. Accessed July 22, 2023. https://www.brookings.edu/articles/how-does-measuring-poverty-and-welfare-affect-american-indian-children

22. Center on Budget and Policy Priorities. *SNAP Helps Millions of Children*; 2017. Accessed January 25, 2023. https://www.cbpp.org/sites/default/files/atoms/files/3-2-17fa2.pdf

23. Center on Budget and Policy Priorities. *SNAP Helps Millions of African Americans*; 2018. Accessed January 25, 2023. https://www.cbpp.org/sites/default/files/atoms/files/3-2-17fa4.pdf

24. Center on Budget and Policy Priorities. *SNAP Helps Millions of Latinos*; 2018. Accessed January 25, 2023. https://www.cbpp.org/sites/default/files/atoms/files/3-2-17fa3.pdf

25. Haley JM, Kenney GM, Bernstein H, Gonzalez D. *One in Five Adults in Immigrant Families With Children Reported Chilling Effects on Public Benefit Receipt in 2019*. Urban Institute; 2020. Accessed January 25, 2023. https://www.urban.org/research/publication/one-five-adults-immigrant-families-children-reported-chilling-effects-public-benefit-receipt-2019

26. Twersky SE. Restrictive state laws aimed at immigrants: effects on enrollment in the food stamp program by U.S. citizen children in immigrant families. *PLoS One*. 2019;14(5):e0215327 PMID: 31042742 doi: 10.1371/journal.pone.0215327

27. Vargas ED, Pirog MA. Mixed-status families and WIC uptake: the effects of risk of deportation on program use. *Soc Sci Q*. 2016;97(3):555–572 PMID: 27642194 doi: 10.1111/ssqu.12286

28. Cohen MS, Schpero WL. Household immigration status had differential impact on Medicaid enrollment in expansion and nonexpansion states. *Health Aff (Millwood)*. 2018;37(3):394–402 PMID: 29505360 doi: 10.1377/hlthaff.2017.0978

29. Guerrero A, Felix Beltran L, Dominguez R, Bustamante A. *Foregoing Healthcare in a Global Pandemic: The Chilling Effects of the Public Charge Rule on Health Access Among Children in California*. UCLA Latino Policy & Politics Initiative; 2021. Accessed January 25, 2023. https://escholarship.org/uc/item/7t28n2kg

30. Gitterman BA, Flanagan PJ, Cotton WH, et al; American Academy of Pediatrics Council on Community Pediatrics. Poverty and child health in the United States. *Pediatrics*. 2016;137(4):e20160339 PMID: 26962238 doi: 10.1542/peds.2016-0339

31. Williams DR, Lawrence JA, Davis BA. Racism and health: evidence and needed research. *Annu Rev Public Health*. 2019;40(1):105–125 PMID: 30601726 doi: 10.1146/annurev-publhealth-040218-043750

32. Boyd RW, Lindo EG, Weeks LD, McLemore MR. On racism: a new standard for publishing on racial health inequities. *Health Aff Forefr*. 2020 doi: 10.1377/forefront.20200630.939347

33. Trent M, Dooley DG, Dougé J, et al; American Academy of Pediatrics Section on Adolescent Health, Council on Community Pediatrics, and Committee on Adolescence. The impact of racism on child and adolescent health. *Pediatrics*. 2019;144(2):e20191765 PMID: 31358665 doi: 10.1542/peds.2019-1765

CHAPTER 3

Implicit and Explicit Biases and the Pediatric Health Professional

Tiffani J. Johnson, MD, MSc

Introduction

The past decade has produced a growing body of research that details the negative impacts of bias and discrimination based on race and other sociodemographic categories, such disability, gender identity, sexual orientation, religion, nationality, language, and socioeconomic status, as well as occurring at the intersection of different categories. This chapter focuses on the effects of implicit and explicit racial biases on children and adolescents in the domains of neighborhoods and housing, education, law enforcement and the carceral system, and health care. Additionally, bias exists in pediatric health workforce diversity, with the effects of these experiences having negative consequences in clinical and academic settings.

Defining and Measuring Bias

- *Explicit biases* are conscious attitudes toward people or groups that can be self-reported.

- *Implicit biases* are attitudes that hover beneath one's consciousness, are activated without an individual's intention or control, and can be influential in one's decision-making and behavior.

The Implicit Association Test (IAT) is a validated instrument used to measure various forms of implicit bias. For example, in the race IAT, participants categorize pictures showing Black and white faces and words representing good and bad constructs (Figure 3–1). Suppose these participants find it easier to perform the stereotypical association of *white* with *good* and *Black* with *bad* (ie, have fewer errors and faster response-latency time) than the counter-stereotypical association of *white* with *bad* and *Black* with *good*. In that case, they have an implicit pro-white/anti-Black bias. Through research using the IAT, we have learned that implicit and explicit biases are related yet distinct mental constructs. For example, individuals can hold one set of conscious beliefs (eg, egalitarianism) in contrast to their implicit beliefs (eg, preference for white people and negative associations with Black people). Moreover, everyone has some type of bias, even when conscious efforts are made toward being unbiased.

Racial bias is a by-product of living in a society in which racism exists at a structural level. Negative associations with the Black race were constructed to justify the enslavement of African people. These associations have been reinforced through *priming*, a

Figure 3-1. Stimuli From the Adult and Child Race Implicit Association Test

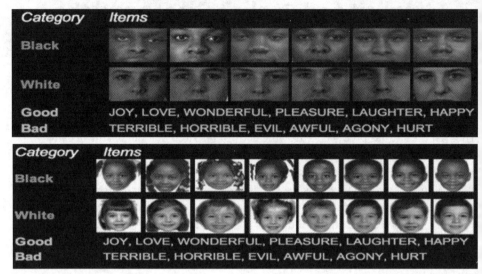

Reproduced from Project Implicit. Take a test. Accessed January 31, 2023. https://implicit.harvard.edu/implicit/takeatest.html.

psychological phenomenon in which stimuli are used to make subconscious connections to our memory. Considering the IAT, implicit associations between Black race and *bad* (and white race and *good*) are rooted in the legacy of white supremacy and reinforced through priming in media, as well as direct and indirect messages received from family, friends, schools, and personal experiences. While it is a less studied area for other populations, data suggest that other minoritized populations (eg, Native American) experience microaggression in the health care arena that can undermine care and affect health outcomes.[1,2]

Child and Adolescent Experiences of Racial Bias

Where They Live: Bias in Neighborhoods and Housing

Children and adolescents who have been racially minoritized are exposed to racial bias across many domains in their lives (Table 3-1). Neighborhoods, for example, are a key social determinant of health. Beyond the documented practice of redlining, implicit and explicit biases contribute to racial discrimination in rental-application screenings,[3] mortgage-lending practices,[4] and appraisals that devalue the houses of Black home owners and neighborhoods.[5] These discriminatory practices influence where children live and contribute to the wealth gap, affecting opportunities over a lifetime. Bias also manifests in neighborhood dynamics, such as the racial profiling and over-policing of Black residents by neighborhood watch organizations.

Where They Learn: Bias in Education

Disparities in suspensions and expulsions have increased attention to bias in the education system. Through the IAT, teachers have demonstrated pro-white/anti-Black implicit racial bias, which may influence their perceptions of Black students as angrier and more dangerous than white peers.[6,7] This bias also manifests as the *adultification* of Black students, who are perceived as older than their peers, resulting in unfair expectations of behaviors and harsher consequences for misbehaviors. Bias is also codified into school policies through dress codes, with disciplinary actions imposed on Black students for wearing hairstyles that are stereotyped as distracting or as promoting gang culture (eg, locs, braids, Afros). These experiences erode trust and a sense of safety while contributing to poorer student-teacher relationships, school engagement, and academic motivation.

Table 3–1. Child and Adolescent Experiences of Racial Bias	
Domain	**Experiences**
Neighborhoods and housing	● Discrimination in rental and mortgage loan applications ● Devaluation of houses of Black home owners and neighborhoods ● Racial profiling by neighborhood watch organizations
Education	● Disparities in educational outcomes (eg, advanced placement, graduation rates) ● Disparities in disciplinary outcomes (eg, suspension, expulsion) ● Teacher interpretation of behavior (eg, "Black boys are dangerous," "Black girls are angry") ● Adultification of Black students ● "School-to-prison" link (ie, funneling minoritized children and adolescents into the juvenile carceral system; refer to Chapter 11, Neurodevelopmental Disorders and the Impact of Racism) ● Policies discriminating against certain hairstyles (eg, locs, braids, Afros).
Law enforcement and the carceral system	● Racial profiling ● Excessive use of force ● Drug policies targeting minoritized groups ● Implicit dehumanization of Black children ● Adultification of children and adolescents who have been accused of crimes or have survived abuse
Health care	● Disparities in clinical care (eg, pain management, child abuse evaluations) ● Disparities in calls to security on patients and their families ● Clinician-patient communication (eg, length of interactions, ratios of talk time [the balance of a clinician's time spent talking with their time spent listening], tone) ● Nonverbal communication with patients (eg, posture, eye contact) ● Stigmatizing language in electronic health records

How Their Rights Are Executed: Bias in Law Enforcement and the Carceral System

Bias plays an important role in racial profiling and child and adolescent experiences during contact with police (refer to Chapter 17, Impact of Interactions With Law Enforcement on the Health of Racially Minoritized Youth). Research has helped illuminate how implicit dehumanization (eg, the association of Black people with apes) is linked with police officers using greater force against Black children relative to children of other races.[8] Similarly, implicit dehumanization is associated with the perception that Black boys, when accused of crimes, are older than their actual ages and more culpable than white peers.[8] Similar bias exists toward Black and Hispanic children who have survived sexual abuse, who are perceived as more responsible for their abuse than their white counterparts.[9]

How They Receive Health Care: Bias in Health Care

Despite striving for equity, health care systems are not immune to bias. For example, physicians explicitly report beliefs about patient intelligence, feelings of affiliation toward a patient, and opinions about risk behaviors and adherence to medical advice that vary on the basis of patient race.[10] Research using the IAT has demonstrated implicit biases in health care that favor white people over Black, Hispanic, and Native American people.[11] Such biases are not limited to views about adults. Clinicians have similar implicit biases against children who are Black, as well as individuals who are gay, who are overweight, or who have disabilities.[11,12] These biases increase when clinicians are experiencing greater cognitive loads, including caring for more patients or working in busy and overcrowded conditions.[13] This finding has been particularly relevant during the ongoing COVID-19 pandemic and respiratory virus surge, with increasing burnout that promotes reliance on heuristics and bias activation.

Many disparities in pediatric health care are driven by bias and stereotyping, including care for sickle cell disease, management of behavioral health emergencies, use of restraints, evaluation of fractures for abuse in young children, and management of pain. For example, pediatricians with greater implicit pro-white/anti-Black bias are more likely to prescribe narcotics for postoperative pain in white children than in Black children.[14] The adultification of Black children in general society is also observed in health care, with Black children being less likely to receive preoperative anxiolysis or have a family member present for anesthesia inductions.[15]

Bias influences patient communication, including length of interactions, ratios of talk time (the balance of a clinician's time spent talking with their time spent listening), and tone. For example, pediatricians are less likely to ask questions of Black children during acute visits than of white children.[16] Bias also influences clinicians' nonverbal communication, in turn influencing attitudes and behaviors during the visit, patient trust, adherence to treatment recommendations, and patient and caregiver satisfaction with care.

Bias is also evident in written communication within the electronic health record (EHR). Examples include language suggesting disbelief of patients' pain, irrelevant descriptors of socioeconomic status, negative stereotypes (eg, "angry," "uncooper ative"), discrediting statements (eg, "claims," "insists," "reportedly"), or using quotations of patients' comments in a mocking manner.[17] Reading stigmatizing language in an EHR is associated with negative attitudes about patients and differences in medical decisions by subsequent clinicians.[17] With increasing patient access to EHRs, stigmatizing language will also erode trust in the patient-clinician relationship.

Pediatric Health Workforce Diversity

Bias also influences pediatric health workforce diversity. For example, pediatric faculty leaders with recruitment roles have demonstrated implicit pro-white/anti-Black bias on a version of the IAT that uses stereotypically Black- and white-sounding names.[18] Bias in the workforce influences interpretations of the achievements of racial and ethnic groups that are underrepresented in medicine (URiM), stereotypes about competence, and labeling of candidates and employees as a flight or failure risk. Gatekeeping often applies a biased and narrow definition of *meritorious*, affecting who enters academia and who and what is published, funded, and promoted. Those who are URiM experience bias in evaluations, grant funding, and research citations while facing a disproportionate burden of service (the diversity tax) and clinical work. As a result, those in groups that are URiM feel pressured to outperform just to be viewed as equally talented as their white peers. These experiences affect workplace climate, job satisfaction, and retention. One of the many benefits of a diverse workforce includes decreased implicit racial bias of medical students, who have positive encounters with faculty members from racial and ethnic groups that are URiM.[19]

Summary

Minoritized children and adolescents are exposed to bias across most social domains, including where they live, where they learn, how their rights are executed, and how they receive health care. Reducing bias requires pediatric health professionals to acknowledge that they exist, be concerned about their consequences, feel motivated to change, and have strategies for replacing biases with responses that are more consistent with their patient-centered goals. In addition, as biases are shaped and reinforced over time through priming, bias-reduction strategies require regular practice so the biases are replaced with new associations that optimize health. Importantly, addressing bias and discrimination requires us to move beyond individual attitudes toward dismantled biased policies and practices within health care systems and society.

Recommendations

Clinical Practice

- To increase awareness of biases, take IATs that are publicly available through Harvard University's Project Implicit (https://implicit.harvard.edu/implicit/takeatest.html) and participate in group discussions about insights gained.

- Complete self-evaluation forms to reflect and monitor progress over time (Figure 3–2).

- Engage in evidence-informed bias-reduction strategies, including perspective taking, stereotype replacement, individuation, exploration of common identities, increased cross-cultural contact, mindfulness, and attentiveness to talk time ratios (Table 3–2).[20]

- Use simulation as a strategy to practice these skills and to reduce the impact of bias on discriminatory behaviors.

Organizations/Systems

- Implement strategies to reduce the number of patients per pediatric health professional to reduce cognitive load.

- Implement pathways for recruitment and holistic review for student and faculty/staff applicants to ensure a diverse pediatric workforce to serve an increasingly diverse population of patients and families.

- Build in breaks during the workday that allow pediatric health professionals to replenish physical and mental resources to reduce cognitive loads and reliance on flawed heuristics such as bias.

- Provide evidence-based guidelines and embedded decision support to reduce clinical uncertainty and bias in decision-making.

- Engage in equity-driven quality improvement efforts that center minoritized groups, engage community voices, and give ongoing and useful feedback to clinicians.

- Develop strategies to increase recruitment and to retain a diverse workforce (refer to Chapter 21, Culturally Congruent Strategies to Build the Pediatric Health Workforce).

- Evaluate policies and procedures with an equity lens, revising them as needed to create a more equitable environment.

Figure 3-2. Clinician Self-evaluation Tool

The following form is intended to help clinicians evaluate their susceptibility toward relying on implicit bias as well as their orientation toward bias mitigation practices. Please answer each question honestly to allow for a holistic evaluation. **In no way is this self-evaluation tool intended for use as a formal metric of a clinician's performance**; instead, it is created for individual use by clinicians seeking to mitigate implicit bias in their patient care practices and increase their capacity for introspection and reflection.

Clinician Self-evaluation Form		Strongly Agree	Agree	Neutral	Strongly Disagree	N/A
Exploring Personal Biases	In the last 6 months, I have taken an Implicit Association Test to explore biases I may possess.					
	I have explored readings and information related to implicit bias in the last 6 months.					
Analyzing Trends	When analyzing treatment and/or care decisions I have made over the last 6 to 12 months, I have NOT noticed any prominent differences in my treatment decisions and/or care provision across identity groups.					
	When analyzing demographic trends of patient feedback over the last 12 months, I have NOT noticed any notable differences in patient perception of care across identity groups.					
Evaluating Practices	In the last 2 weeks of care provision, I have been attentive to the talk time ratios—the balance of time spent talking with vs. listening to—with patients of various backgrounds.					
	Reflecting on my most recent 15 patients, I have consistently sought to connect with my patients around our common identity/ies.					
	Reflecting on my most recent 15 patients, I have actively engaged in perspective-taking when providing care to my patients. *Perspective-taking* refers to the imagining of the experiences, feelings and thinking of one's patients to build empathy and understanding.					
	Over the last 6 months, I have frequently engaged in practices aimed at increasing my cognitive control (eg, mindfulness meditation) in an effort to mitigate the influence of implicit bias in my care provision.					
	Institutional Leaders: I have made intentional decisions to construct diverse clinical care teams and facilitate intergroup contact over the last 3 months.					

N/A indicates not applicable.

This form is made available with permission from The Kirwan Institute for the Study of Race and Ethnicity.

Table 3–2. Strategies for Pediatric Health Professionals to Confront Personal Biases

Strategy	Description
Perspective taking	• Consciously assess situations from the point of view of caregivers, patients, colleagues, and community members who come from a background (eg, race, socioeconomic status, sexual orientation) different from your own. • For example, when experiencing a challenging patient or family interaction, try to take a moment to consider what biases you bring to the scenario and think about the encounter from their perspective. Consider what barriers they may face when navigating the health care system or how past experiences in health care and general society might influence their attitudes, behaviors, and communication styles during the encounter. The best way to do so is by respectfully asking instead of making assumptions.
Stereotype replacement	• Practice recognizing and labeling stereotyping when it occurs (eg, "Black boys are violent," "Black girls are angry," "Hispanic children are illegal immigrants"). • Use counter-stereotypical imaging by imagining individuals such as public figures or friends whose traits contrast stereotypes typically associated with a group. • Focus on replacing stereotypes when they come up and avoiding them in future interactions with minoritized groups.
Individuation	• Try to get to know patients and colleagues on a more personal level, allowing yourself to focus on their personal characteristics instead of their group-based characteristics, which can often be influenced by bias and stereotypes. • Seek to gain greater understanding of the complexity and nuances of their experiences as an individual beyond the demographic groups they belong to. • This strategy should not be confused with a color-blind ideology, in which one claims or seeks to not see race. Instead, pediatric health professionals should have a color consciousness that values the experiences and worldviews of different groups while recognizing that these experiences are not a monolith.
Exploration of common identities	• When taking time to get to know individuals on the basis of their personal characteristics, try to connect with them over shared interests to help reduce in-group vs out-group thinking.

Table 3–2 (*continued*)	
Strategy	**Description**

Increased cross-cultural contact	● Seek opportunities to authentically and respectfully engage with people and groups from backgrounds different from your own.
	● Be cautious to not engage in cultural voyeurism, or objectifying or exploiting others' cultures.
	● Take time to listen, reflect, and understand during these encounters.
	● For example,
	  • Visit and support minority-owned businesses.
	  • Attend services for a religion different from your own.
	  • Attend events such as cultural heritage festivals or LGBTQ+ pride activities. Spend time learning about the history of the event, and consider supporting the event through volunteering or donating to prevent an unequal exchange, in which you are taking without giving.
	  • Go to a park in a different community, and consider volunteering for a park cleanup.
	  • Attend an academic meeting that is sponsored by an organization representing the interests of an underrepresented group, such as the National Medical Association (www.nmanet.org) or the National Hispanic Medical Association (www.nhmamd.org).

Mindfulness	● Being present in the moment to increase awareness of your thoughts, emotions, and environment ● Often practiced through meditation, which is widely available through phone apps ● Helps slow down thinking processes and increase intent to reduce automatic reactions and fear responses ● Can increase empathy and compassion
Attentiveness to talk time ratios	● Pay attention to how much time is spent listening to patients and their caregivers instead of talking to them or at them.

References

1. Walls ML, Gonzalez J, Gladney T, Onello E. Unconscious biases: racial microaggressions in American Indian health care. *J Am Board Fam Med.* 2015;28(2):231–239 PMID: 25748764 doi: 10.3122/jabfm.2015.02.140194

2. Maina IW, Belton TD, Ginzberg S, Singh A, Johnson TJ. A decade of studying implicit racial/ethnic bias in healthcare providers using the Implicit Association Test. *Soc Sci Med.* 2018;199:219–229 PMID: 28532892 doi: 10.1016/j.socscimed.2017.05.009

3. Rosen E, Garboden PME, Cossyleon JE. Racial discrimination in housing: how landlords use algorithms and home visits to screen tenants. *Am Sociol Rev.* 2021;86(5):787–822 doi: 10.1177/00031224211029618

4. Hanson A, Hawley Z, Martin H, Liu B. Discrimination in mortgage lending: evidence from a correspondence experiment. *J Urban Econ.* 2016;92:48–65 doi: 10.1016/j.jue.2015.12.004

5. Howell J, Korver-Glenn E. Neighborhoods, race, and the twenty-first-century housing appraisal industry. *Sociol Race Ethn (Thousand Oaks).* 2018;4(4):473–490 doi: 10.1177/2332649218755178

6. Blackson EA, Gerdes M, Segan E, Anokam C, Johnson TJ. Racial bias toward children in the early childhood education setting. *J Early Child Res.* 2022;20(3):277–292 doi: 10.1177/1476718X221087051

7. Halberstadt AG, Castro VL, Chu Q, Lozada FT, Sims CM. Preservice teachers' racialized emotion recognition, anger bias, and hostility attributions. *Contemp Educ Psychol.* 2018;54:125–138 doi: 10.1016/j.cedpsych.2018.06.004

8. Goff PA, Jackson MC, Di Leone BAL, Culotta CM, DiTomasso NA. The essence of innocence: consequences of dehumanizing Black children. *J Pers Soc Psychol.* 2014;106(4):526–545 PMID: 24564373 doi: 10.1037/a0035663

9. Bottoms BL, Davis SL, Epstein MA. Effect of victim and defendant race on jurors' decisions in child sex abuse cases. *J Appl Soc Psychol.* 2004;34(1):1–33 doi: 10.1111/j.1559-1816.2004.tb02535.x

10. van Ryn M, Burke J. The effect of patient race and socio-economic status on physicians' perceptions of patients. *Soc Sci Med.* 2000;50(6):813–828 PMID: 10695979 doi: 10.1016/S0277-9536(99)00338-X

11. Maina IW, Belton TD, Ginzberg S, Singh A, Johnson TJ. A decade of studying implicit racial/ethnic bias in healthcare providers using the Implicit Association Test. *Soc Sci Med.* 2018;199:219–229 PMID: 28532892 doi: 10.1016/j.socscimed.2017.05.009

12. Johnson TJ, Winger DG, Hickey RW, et al. Comparison of physician implicit racial bias toward adults versus children. *Acad Pediatr.* 2017;17(2):120–126 PMID: 27620844 doi: 10.1016/j.acap.2016.08.010

13. Johnson TJ, Hickey RW, Switzer GE, et al. The impact of cognitive stressors in the emergency department on physician implicit racial bias. *Acad Emerg Med.* 2016;23(3):297–305 PMID: 26763939 doi: 10.1111/acem.12901

14. Sabin JA, Greenwald AG. The influence of implicit bias on treatment recommendations for 4 common pediatric conditions: pain, urinary tract infection, attention deficit hyperactivity disorder, and asthma. *Am J Public Health.* 2012;102(5):988–995 PMID: 22420817 doi: 10.2105/AJPH.2011.300621

15. Baetzel A, Brown DJ, Koppera P, Rentz A, Thompson A, Christensen R. Adultification of Black children in pediatric anesthesia. *Anesth Analg.* 2019;129(4):1118–1123 PMID: 31295177 doi: 10.1213/ANE.0000000000004274

16. Stivers T, Majid A. Questioning children: interactional evidence of implicit bias in medical interviews. *Soc Psychol Q.* 2007;70(4):424–441 doi: 10.1177/019027250707000410

17. Goddu A, O'Conor KJ, Lanzkron S, et al. Do words matter? stigmatizing language and the transmission of bias in the medical record. *J Gen Intern Med.* 2018;33(5):685–691 PMID: 29374357 doi: 10.1007/s11606-017-4289-2

18. Johnson TJ, Ellison AM, Dalembert G, et al. Implicit bias in pediatric academic medicine. *J Natl Med Assoc.* 2017;109(3):156–163 PMID: 28987244

19. van Ryn M, Hardeman R, Phelan SM, et al. Medical school experiences associated with change in implicit racial bias among 3547 students: a medical student CHANGES study report. *J Gen Intern Med.* 2015;30(12):1748–1756 PMID: 26129779 doi: 10.1007/s11606-015-3447-7

20. Johnson TJ. Racial bias and its impact on children and adolescents. *Pediatr Clin North Am.* 2020;67(2):425–436 PMID: 32122570 doi: 10.1016/j.pcl.2019.12.011

How Adults Can Promote Positive Racial and Ethnic Identities in the Context of Structural Racism

Diane L. Hughes, PhD, and Valerie N. Adams-Bass, PhD

Introduction

The 21st century has been marked by broad recognition of historical and contemporary racism against people of color in almost every aspect of American life, including where people live, how much they earn, what their health status is, which schools they attend, and what access they have to opportunities. Discrimination against people of color at the individual and interpersonal levels has increased. In 2021, the FBI reported the highest number of hate crimes in 12 years: 65% were based on race, ethnicity, or ancestry.[1] New insight into the magnitude and persistence of racism in the United States resulted in calls from Fortune 500 CEOs, university presidents, professional organizations, and others for a change in policies and practices to reduce racial oppression. Rochelle Walensky, the director of the Centers for Disease Control and Prevention, declared racism a public health threat, as did 20 states and 33 cities across the United States.[2,3]

As more individuals and institutions acknowledge structural racism and discrimination, adults who care for youth (children and adolescents) need information about how youth react to these phenomena and need strategies to help youth navigate and dismantle persistent racial injustice and inequality. Developmental science offers evidence-based knowledge in this realm. Parents and caregivers, pediatric health professionals, and others can look to racial socialization research to identify effective strategies by which to ground guidance for supporting youth as they navigate the challenges of racism in the United States. *Racial socialization* is "the process through which parents [or caregivers] and other socializing agents communicate these filtered messages to youth about the significance of race."[4]

Racial Learning

Racial learning is the process through which youth negotiate, interpret, and make meaning of the various and often conflicting messages they receive about race.[5] Early in development, children naturally notice and make meaning of race, regardless of whether others label the construct or have conversations with the children about it.[6] Phenotypic differences associated with racial group membership (eg, skin color, hair type, clothing, language) are perceptually salient and impossible to overlook.

Eye-tracking studies have shown that infants notice and pay attention to race by the time they are 3 to 6 months of age.[7] Perceptual salience is followed by other cognitive and social processes that prompt youth to form attitudes and beliefs about racial differences. For example, in preschool, children use race as a basis for questioning and including/excluding other children.[8] By kindergarten, they show in-group preference and racial bias.[9] By the age of 10 years, they understand that people can hold and act on racial stereotypes. They also understand unfair treatment and report their own experiences with bias and discrimination.[10] Thus, perceptual and other cognitive processes contribute to their racial attitudes and beliefs.

External forces and environmental conditions shape what youth learn about race, mainly because they grow up with race as a stratifying category. They are also exposed to racial inequities in income, neighborhood quality, education, familial and personal health statuses, and illness and death.[11] Further, messages about race are embedded within the observed racial disparities in who is affected by school suspensions, who enrolls in honors rather than general classes, and who is most likely to live in affluent neighborhoods rather than modest- or low-income housing. Places of worship, family social networks, neighborhoods, schools, classrooms, and extracurricular activities are often racially segregated, a separation giving meaning to status in the context of racial group membership. Youth notice, interpret, and learn race from the racial patterns and regularities they observe in society.[12] Thus, caregivers and pediatric health professionals should make space for youth to unpack and interpret these oppressive structures in ways that support their actions to cope with, resist, and dismantle them.

Racial Socialization

While youth develop racial attitudes and beliefs as part of the typical developmental processes, adults act as powerful protectors who can filter racial bias through an alternative, more positive reframed lens. Although many individuals (eg, teachers, coaches, peers, community members) convey messages about race, the most salient research on racial socialization focuses on the role of parents and caregivers. The sections that follow describe the 2 types of socialization studied most: promoting positive racial and ethnic identities in youth and protecting youth against racism and discrimination.

Promoting Positive Racial and Ethnic Identities in Youth

Developing a positive racial identity is a fundamental task for youth in the United States, especially those from groups that have been racially minoritized, subsequently referred to as *minoritized youth* for ease of reading. Racial identity has become a part of a social identity based on racial group membership.[13] Between childhood and adolescence, most youth develop a positive racial identity that includes favorable attitudes, feelings of group pride and belonging, and an increasingly clear perspective on race's role in their self-views. Youth with more positive racial identities also report better adjustment, including better social, psychological, academic, behavioral, and relational adjustment.[14]

Caregivers and other adults who work with youth play a crucial role in promoting and supporting their positive racial identities through *cultural socialization*, which involves practices that (1) teach youth about cultural heritage, ancestry, and history; (2) maintain and promote cultural customs and traditions; and (3) instill cultural, racial, and ethnic pride.[15] For instance, many parents and caregivers of color intentionally try to bolster a child's feelings of attachment to their racial group, to ensure the internalization of positive cultural values and beliefs, and to deeply ground the child in their group's history and heritage, beginning at an early age. Activities may include participating in cultural celebrations, visiting museums, reading books about historical figures and events, and having representative toys, books, magazines, and art in the home. Youth of parents/caregivers who practice more frequent cultural socialization explore their identities earlier and more often than their counterparts. They also show more positive attitudes about their race and view it as a central part of their identity. Associations between cultural socialization and racial identity have been found across racial and ethnic groups and developmental stages from preschool through emerging adulthood.[16] Research suggests that adults' cultural socialization messages benefit children because these messages focus on group strengths and foster knowledge and skills that youth use to manage racialized encounters as they navigate the world.

Protecting Youth Against Racism and Discrimination

Minoritized youth routinely report exposure to racial discrimination from various individuals (eg, peers, teachers, and store owners) and across multiple settings (eg, school, neighborhood, and extracurricular programs). Discrimination can be a negative, stressful, toxic, and traumatic experience for youth. Experiencing it more frequently has been associated with a catalog of adjustment indicators, including poorer grades, increased anxiety and depression, diminished psychological well-being, poorer relationships with peers and adults, lower sense of school belonging, lower likelihood of college completion, decreased emotion regulation, higher anger, vigilance, risk-taking behaviors, disrupted sleep, unhealthy cortisol levels, cellular inflammation, and hippocampal volume.[17]

Given the harm that discrimination causes, caregivers and pediatric health professionals need the skills to support minoritized youth through these experiences. However, discussions can be sensitive and are often riddled with complexity. Caregivers may be uncomfortable and may find it challenging to discuss racial discrimination or support youth following discriminatory experiences. One study showed that youth of color rarely disclose their experiences of discrimination with their parents/caregivers because they expect negative parental reactions or want to protect their parents/caregivers from worrying about them.[18] Table 4–1 summarizes 3 intervention projects that have empirically evaluated the effects of programs designed to increase skill and effectiveness of parents and caregivers in discussing racial intolerance and injustice with their youth.

Table 4–1. Racial and Ethnic Socialization Programs for Parents and Caregivers	
Program Title	**Program Components**
Engaging, Managing, and Bonding through Race (EMBRace)[a]	● Culturally based therapeutic intervention ● Designed for Black youth aged 10–14 y and their caregivers ● Focuses on enhancing Black youth's and families' capacity to confront racial stress and trauma together
Talking About Race[b]	● Customized for caregivers to explore strategies for addressing race and racism with their youth ● Educates on how children perceive race, provides skills for engaging in age-appropriate conversations with a racial equity lens ● Offers opportunities to practice strategies that promote positive racial identity development
One Talk at a Time[c]	● Uses video-based role modeling and coaching to increase caregivers' readiness and efficacy for effective, open, and helpful conversations with youth about race and racism

[a] Anderson RE, McKenny M, Mitchell A, Koku L, Stevenson HC. EMBRacing racial stress and trauma: preliminary feasibility and coping responses of a racial socialization intervention. *J Black Psychol.* 2018;44(1):25–46.
[b] Center for Racial Justice in Education. Our services. Accessed January 30, 2023. https://centerracialjustice.org/our-services.
[c] Stein GL, Coard SI, Gonzalez LM, Kiang L, Sircar JK. One talk at a time: developing an ethnic-racial socialization intervention for Black, Latinx, and Asian American families. *J Soc Issues.* 2021;77(4):1014–1036.

Recommendations on How Pediatric Health Professionals Can Support Youth and Families

Professionals in the pediatric community are core members of the nexus of adults who ensure youth's positive physical and mental health. In this role, we need to position ourselves to effectively support their positive racial identities and to prepare them to recognize and resist the negative racial dynamics to which they are exposed. Following are some examples of steps we can take to begin this process:

● Pediatric health professionals and others can begin by examining their own biases, assumptions about race, and comfort levels. Harvard University's Project Implicit can be a useful resource to begin this process (https://implicit.harvard.edu/implicit/takeatest.html). Map your social network to examine areas of diversity within it. Study your home for things suggesting that you value diversity. Pay attention to how you feel and behave when you encounter injustice or unfairness as a bystander or in the media.

● Youth and caregivers need to feel welcome and safe in the places they go. Examine the physical and architectural space in which you meet with youth and families for representation of diverse racial and ethnic and other groups. Posters, magazines, signage, and staff diversity can support positive youth racial identities.

● Ask parents and caregivers what they want their youth to think about race or about managing group differences. Assure them that talking with youth about race is desirable; it will not make them racist or encourage them to notice race when they would not otherwise have. Also, encourage parents and caregivers to answer rather than avoid or redirect young people's questions about race.

● Look for opportunities to probe youth for their own experiences with racial bias and discrimination. Listen to and validate youth experiences without judgment.

● Encourage parents and caregivers to bring diversity into their youth's lives by having diverse toys, games, and books in the home; by introducing them to people with diverse cultures; and by taking them to places with diverse cultural experiences.

Summary

● Historical and contemporary racism affects the lives of people of color, including youth.

● Racial learning is a process that youth learn from caregivers and other adults in their lives.

● Racial socialization is an active process that can be protective.

● Adults should prepare youth to manage structural racism and discrimination.

● Professional organizations should provide recommendations and opportunities for pediatric health professionals to bolster their knowledge and skills to support the health and well-being of youth of color.

References

1. Equal Justice Initiative. FBI reports hate crimes at highest level in 12 years. September 9, 2021. Accessed January 30, 2023. https://eji.org/news/fbi-reports-hate-crimes-at-highest-level-in-12-years

2. Media statement from CDC director Rochelle P. Walensky, MD, MPH, on racism and health. News release. Centers for Disease Control and Prevention; April 8, 2021. Accessed January 30, 2023. https://www.cdc.gov/media/releases/2021/s0408-racism-health.html

3. American Public Health Association. Racism is a public health crisis. Accessed January 30, 2023. https://www.apha.org/topics-and-issues/health-equity/racism-and-health/racism-declarations

4. Hughes DL, Watford JA, Del Toro J. A transactional/ecological perspective on ethnic-racial identity, socialization, and discrimination. *Adv Child Dev Behav.* 2016;51:1–41 PMID: 27474421 doi: 10.1016/bs.acdb.2016.05.001

5. Winkler EN. *Learning Race, Learning Place: Shaping Racial Identities and Ideas in African American Childhoods.* Rutgers University Press; 2012

6. Bigler RS, Liben LS. Developmental intergroup theory: explaining and reducing children's social stereotyping and prejudice. *Curr Dir Psychol Sci.* 2007;16(3):162–166 doi: 10.1111/j.1467-8721.2007.00496.x

7. Kelly DJ, Quinn PC, Slater AM, et al. Three-month-olds, but not newborns, prefer own-race faces. *Dev Sci.* 2005;8(6):F31–F36 PMID: 16246233 doi: 10.1111/j.1467-7687.2005.0434a.x

8. Feagin JR, Van Ausdale D. *The First R: How Children Learn Race and Racism.* Rowman & Littlefield Publishers; 2001

9. Baron AS, Banaji MR. The development of implicit attitudes: evidence of race evaluations from ages 6 and 10 and adulthood. *Psychol Sci.* 2006;17(1):53–58 PMID: 16371144 doi: 10.1111/j.1467-9280.2005.01664.x

10. McKown C. Age and ethnic variation in children's thinking about the nature of racism. *J Appl Dev Psychol.* 2004;25(5):597–617 doi: 10.1016/j.appdev.2004.08.001

11. NCHS data on racial and ethnic disparities. Fact sheet. National Center for Health Statistics. March 2019. Accessed January 30, 2023. https://www.cdc.gov/nchs/data/factsheets/factsheet_disparities.htm

12. Hughes DL, Watford JA. Racial regularities: setting-level dynamics as a source of ethnic-racial socialization. *Am J Community Psychol.* 2022;70(1–2):3–17 doi: 10.1002/ajcp.12565

13. Rivas-Drake D, Seaton EK, Markstrom C, et al; Ethnic and Racial Identity in the 21st Century Study Group. Ethnic and racial identity in adolescence: implications for psychosocial, academic, and health outcomes. *Child Dev.* 2014;85(1):40–57 PMID: 24490891 doi: 10.1111/cdev.12200

14. Rivas-Drake D, Syed M, Umaña-Taylor A, et al; Ethnic and Racial Identity in the 21st Century Study Group. Feeling good, happy, and proud: a meta-analysis of positive ethnic-racial affect and adjustment. *Child Dev.* 2014;85(1):77–102 PMID: 24490893 doi: 10.1111/cdev.12175

15. Hughes D, Chen L. The nature of parents' race-related communications to children: a developmental perspective. In: Balter L, Tamis-LeMonda CS, eds. *Child Psychology: A Handbook of Contemporary Issues.* Psychology Press; 1999:467–490

16. Huguley JP, Wang MT, Vasquez AC, Guo J. Parental ethnic-racial socialization practices and the construction of children of color's ethnic-racial identity: a research synthesis and meta-analysis. *Psychol Bull.* 2019;145(5):437–458 PMID: 30896188 doi: 10.1037/bul0000187

17. Trent M, Dooley DG, Dougé J, et al; American Academy of Pediatrics Section on Adolescent Health, Council on Community Pediatrics, and Committee on Adolescence. The impact of racism on child and adolescent health. *Pediatrics.* 2019;144(2):e2019191765

18. Juang LP, Syed M. Sharing stories of discrimination with parents. *J Adolesc.* 2014;37(3):303–312 doi: 10.1016/j.adolescence.2014.02.004

CHAPTER 5

Understanding Racism and Adolescence

Anisha Abraham, MD, MPH, and Maria Trent, MD, MPH

Introduction

Racism is a system of oppression that categorizes and stratifies people into "races" and creates adverse childhood experiences in which the healthy development and well-being of adolescents and families are undermined through differential treatment that leads to social disadvantage.[1] Pervasive racism exists in societies around the globe, but it has been so distinctly codified into the American experience that it has been identified as a US public health emergency.[2]

Experiences of racism, particularly if internalized, can influence self-esteem, risk-taking behaviors, and the emotional well-being of adolescents and young adults.[3,4] The adolescent brain continues to develop, with modifications of brain networks that leverage life experiences, until the age of 25 years. Adolescent development also includes physical, gender and sexual, and cultural and ethnic identities. The development of cultural identity can be challenging for adolescents who must reconcile more than one culture or must reconcile other forms of intersectionality in their lives. There can be strengths and challenges to multiculturalism, which have emerged from domestic and global research about adolescents.

Pediatric health professionals, parents and caregivers, and others who work with adolescents need to be sensitive to teenage development, including the important role of racial socialization as a mediator for their experiences of racism, and need to foster positive identity development.[5] Early intervention through screening before adolescence, conversations that recognize and acknowledge unique injustices faced during adolescence, and thoughtful scaffolding by caregivers can help adolescents navigate and counter the negative physical, emotional, and social effects of racism as they approach autonomy.

Why Adolescence Is Such a Critical Period

During adolescence, the physical, cognitive, and emotional transformations result in important growth opportunities as adolescents gradually move toward autonomy. Early in adolescence, identity development peaks as adolescents begin to acutely notice their differences from others while feeling a tremendous need to belong. Pulling away from family to establish independence is an important step, allowing adolescents to assume natural risks associated with embracing new challenges such as trying out for sports, learning how to drive, navigating communication with teachers and coaches, building romantic relationships, and leaving home. The experiences and lessons learned by tackling these developmental milestones rewire the adolescent brain, inspiring adolescents to seek novelty, even in the face of unfamiliar and occasionally unadvisable pursuits, as they approach full development. Research shows that the brains of children and adolescents are more sensitive to stress than the brains of adults and that chronic stress is damaging to areas of the brain that control reactions to stress and regulate mood, growth, body temperature, and sexuality. Although some level of stress is beneficial and unavoidable during adolescence, ongoing daily stress from preventable causes can disrupt healthy brain development and increase the risk for mental health issues.[6]

Fortunately, adolescents are better learners because their brain cells have greater adaptability, which allows them to gain new skills. Thus, the adolescent brain is vulnerable to stress yet highly adaptable to learning.

Identity Development

A key developmental milestone during adolescence is identity development. Identity incorporates an individual's unique personality, sense of purpose and abilities, and connection to others, but it is also shaped by the perception of oneself within a family, a culture, and a community. The tension between the biological changes in adolescents and their cognitive development is essential for a successful transition to young adulthood. As discussed in Chapter 9, The Intersection of Race, Sexuality, and Gender Identity During Adolescence, adolescents begin to incorporate the meaning of physical appearance, race and ethnicity, religion, nationality, and sexual orientation and gender identity as their worldviews shift and moral systems develop. An adolescent can also feel and experience differential treatment because of their age and other identities. Without an ability to see, name, oppose, and replace adversity arising just as their individual identity is forming, they can experience assaults on their psyche and well-being as they move into adulthood (refer to Chapter 28, Helping Minoritized Youth Resist Racism).

The Importance of Belonging

There is a critical need for each adolescent to create safe spaces with peers in which their identity is accepted, reinforced, and valued as they tackle the typical challenges of emerging autonomy.[7] When adolescents experience uncertainty or feel vulnerable, their peers will help refine operational identities as their outer circumstances potentially shift. Research consistently demonstrates that adolescents who develop a positive sense of racial identity by young adulthood experience less biological health and risk-related adversity. For example, they may perform better academically, engage more civically, truly value diversity as adults, and engage less in substance use, violent behavior, and high-risk sexual activity. Also, those who can build effective relationships across differences are ultimately more resilient and more able to successfully navigate a multicultural world.[8,9]

Impact of Exposure on Adolescent Development, Risk-taking, and Long-term Health

Racism, Education, and Wages

Exposure to racism can occur at home, in school, and in other areas of an adolescent's community. These exposures may result from structural barriers that have been created over time to acts of racism that are personally mediated, including implicit biases, microaggressions, and macroaggressions. Although parents and caregivers may be able to shield younger children, adolescents become acutely aware of the differences in their everyday experiences and in their access to the basics of daily living. Further, as adolescents age, it substantially increases their risk of encountering other adolescents and adults who harbor negative stereotypes and prejudices about their racial and ethnic identities.

Racism affects the quality of adolescents' lives, from where they reside, to their education, to the safety of where they play. Most individuals understand that a community's tax base often defines these entities; however, few understand that race-based limitations on where people live, and the value of their communities (known as *redlining*) that is codified in federal policy, effectively segregated the United States and compounded substantial wealth and educational gaps over time.[10] The spiral from related inequality within the education system and over-policing in under-resourced, segregated schools lead to community underemployment, low wages, disproportionate rates of incarceration, and poorer overall health. Police interactions alone have been demonstrated to negatively affect emotional well-being and risk-taking behaviors of youth aged 9 to 26 years.[11]

Racism and Mental Health Status

As described further in Chapter 12, Addressing the Impact of Racism on the Mental Health of Youth: A Focus on Pediatric Health Professionals, experiences of racism correlate with poorer mental health, including depression, anxiety, and psychological stress, as well as decreased physical health.[12,13] Social belonging, or an intrinsic need during adolescence, can be disrupted by experiences of discrimination. A recent study among an ethnically diverse sample of adolescents who completed measures of ethnic and nonethnic discrimination, sleep, loneliness, and stress demonstrated that Asian American, Black, and Latinx[a] students who experienced any discrimination also experienced reduced sleep quality and greater loneliness. Nonethnic discrimination was further associated with perceived stress.[14]

---

[a] In this chapter, we use *Latinx* when referring to people of Latin American origin or descent as a whole. It is a gender-neutral and gender-inclusive alternative to *Latino*. For a brief history of this term, including a rationale, refer to the book introduction.

Although socioeconomic status can serve as a protective factor against racism, emerging data from research with Black adolescents suggest that those who have educated parents (a proxy for higher socioeconomic status) report higher rates of depressive symptoms, raising concerns about the experiences they have navigating educational and other community environments with limited diversity.[15] Although racial and other forms of discrimination are not limited to the United States, they have been woven into the fabric of American history. The American Academy of Pediatrics[16] and researchers and child advocates around the globe have started to examine the impact of race on health and well-being and are making similar observations.[17]

Adolescent/Family/Community Empowerment Strategies to Optimize Development

The American Academy of Pediatrics recommends that parents, pediatric health professionals, and caregivers engage in proactive work to help adolescents develop a positive identity (Table 5–1). Also, parents and caregivers should use a structured approach to raising resisters (refer to Chapter 28, Helping Minoritized Youth Resist Racism) in an evolving sociopolitical landscape in which formation of identity and discussions of racism and equity have become controversial yet incidents of racial discrimination continue to be public but largely unchecked by society at large. It is critical that pediatric health and other adolescent-serving professionals engage in behaviors designed to both prevent and intervene on experiences of racism during adolescence to reduce their impact on healthy development and well-being during emerging adulthood.

Summary

Adolescents are uniquely affected by experiences of discrimination because they are vulnerable to assaults as they grow to adult size and they have not yet solidified their evolving identity. It is therefore essential that adolescent-serving professionals be prepared to work with adolescents and families to ensure prosocial perspectives on their evolving racial and ethnic identities so stereotyping and prejudice do not physically or emotionally harm them. Trusted adults must also listen to adolescents, help them understand and name their experiences appropriately, oppose incidents of racism without creating more harm, and try to replace these adverse experiences with affirming ones. Communities and institutions must adapt to ensure that the social safety nets for adolescents allow for safe exploration of identity while encouraging diverse and inclusive school and social environments.

Table 5–1. Prevention and Intervention Strategies for Pediatric Health Professionals to Use When Working With Adolescents Experiencing Racial or Other Forms of Discrimination	
Prevention Strategies	**Intervention Strategies**
<ul><li>Encourage parents and caregivers to teach adolescents about race and ethnicity to prepare adolescents for a racialized world.</li><li>Discuss the value of diversity and inclusion.</li><li>Create alone time within the visit for them to openly share.</li><li>Ask how they are managing their school and community experiences.</li><li>Ask about their evolving identity to understand their intersecting identities.</li><li>Listen to their stories about everyday experiences that shape identity and self-esteem.</li><li>Include queries about peer experiences and differential or unfair treatment.</li><li>Be honest about history, because they have access to the internet.</li></ul>	<ul><li>Listen by using core principles of patient-centered communication, leading with empathy and partnership while avoiding judgment and victim blaming.</li><li>Be prepared to offer strategic advice to patients and families through a strength-based "raising resisters" approach (refer to Chapter 28, Helping Minoritized Youth Resist Racism).[a]<ul><li>Read/see it.</li><li>Name it.</li><li>Oppose it.</li><li>Replace it.</li></ul></li><li>Activate parents and caregivers with adolescent knowledge and consent.</li><li>Cultivate resources to support them in the community.</li><li>Consider behavioral health services.</li><li>Arrange a follow-up to reassess issues while leaving the door open for them to return for new challenges.</li></ul>

[a] Ward JV. *The Skin We're In: Teaching Our Teens to Be Emotionally Strong, Socially Smart, and Spiritually Connected.* Fireside; 2000.

References

1. Priest N, Doery K, Truong M, et al. Updated systematic review and meta-analysis of studies examining the relationship between reported racism and health and well-being for children and youth: a protocol. *BMJ Open.* 2021;11(6):e043722 doi: 10.1136/bmjopen-2020-043722

2. Vestal C. Racism is a public health crisis, say cities and counties. Stateline. June 15, 2020. Accessed January 31, 2023. https://www.pewtrusts.org/en/research-and-analysis/blogs/stateline/2020/06/15/racism-is-a-public-health-crisis-say-cities-and-counties

3. Priest N, Paradies Y, Trenerry B, et al. A systematic review of studies examining the relationship between reported racism and health and wellbeing for children and young people. *Soc Sci Med.* 2013;95:115–127 PMID: 23312306 doi: 10.1016/j.socscimed.2012.11.031

4. James D. Internalized racism and past-year major depressive disorder among African-Americans: the role of ethnic identity and self-esteem. *J Racial Ethn Health Disparities.* 2017;4(4):659–670 PMID: 27444489 doi: 10.1007/s40615-016-0269-1

5. Stevenson HC, Arrington EG. Racial/ethnic socialization mediates perceived racism and the racial identity of African American adolescents. *Cultur Divers Ethnic Minor Psychol.* 2009;15(2):125–136 PMID: 19364199 doi: 10.1037/a0015500

6. Echouffo-Tcheugui JB, Conner SC, Himali JJ, et al. Circulating cortisol and cognitive and structural brain measures: the Framingham Heart Study. *Neurology.* 2018;91(21):e1961–e1970 PMID: 30355700 doi: 10.1212/WNL.0000000000006549

7. Tatum BD. *Why Are All the Black Kids Sitting Together in the Cafeteria? and Other Conversations About Race.* Basic Books; 2017

8. Wells AS, Fox L, Cordova-Cobo D. How racially diverse schools and classrooms can benefit all students. The Century Foundation. February 9, 2016. Accessed January 31, 2023. https://tcf.org/content/report/how-racially-diverse-schools-and-classrooms-can-benefit-all-students

9. Kamenetz A. The evidence that white children benefit from integrated schools. NPR Ed. October 19, 2015. Accessed January 31, 2023. https://www.npr.org/sections/ed/2015/10/19/446085513/the-evidence-that-white-children-benefit-from-integrated-schools

10. Rothstein R. *The Color of Law: A Forgotten History of How Our Government Segregated America.* Liveright; 2017

11. Jindal M, Mistry KB, Trent M, McRae A, Thornton RLJ. Police exposures and the health and well-being of Black youth in the US: a systematic review. *JAMA Pediatr.* 2022;176(1):78–88 PMID: 34491292 doi: 10.1001/jamapediatrics.2021.2929

12. Paradies Y, Ben J, Denson N, et al. Racism as a determinant of health: a systematic review and meta-analysis. *PLoS One.* 2015;10(9):e0138511 doi: 10.1371/journal.pone.0138511

13. Cheadle JE, Goosby BJ, Jochman JC, Tomaso CC, Kozikowski Yancey CB, Nelson TD. Race and ethnic variation in college students' allostatic regulation of racism-related stress. *Proc Natl Acad Sci USA.* 2020;117(49):31053–31062 PMID: 33229568 doi: 10.1073/pnas.1922025117

14. Majeno A, Tsai KM, Huynh VW, McCreath H, Fuligni AJ. Discrimination and sleep difficulties during adolescence: the mediating roles of loneliness and perceived stress. *J Youth Adolesc.* 2018;47(1):135–147 PMID: 29164378 doi: 10.1007/s10964-017-0755-8

15. Cheng ER, Cohen A, Goodman E. The role of perceived discrimination during childhood and adolescence in understanding racial and socioeconomic influences on depression in young adulthood. *J Pediatr.* 2015;166(2):370–7.e1 PMID: 25454941 doi: 10.1016/j.jpeds.2014.10.010

16. Trent M, Dooley DG, Dougé J, et al; American Academy of Pediatrics Section on Adolescent Health, Council on Community Pediatrics and Committee on Adolescence. The impact of racism on child and adolescent health. *Pediatrics.* 2019;144(2):e20191765 PMID: 31358665 doi: 10.1542/peds.2019-1765

17. Olusanya BO. Systemic racism in global health: a personal reflection. *Lancet Glob Health.* 2021;9(8):e1051–e1052 PMID: 34297951 doi: 10.1016/S2214-109X(21)00147-9

Part 2. Intersections of Racism and Health for Children and Adolescents

Section 1. Population-Specific Issues

CHAPTER 6

Considering Multiracial Youth: Identity Challenges and Health Outcomes

Brenda Straka, PhD, and Sarah Gaither, PhD

Introduction

There are overarching and well-documented health disparities between racial majority and minority groups. Yet, the Multiracial population, or those claiming membership to more than one racial group, has been largely excluded from health disparity research. This dearth of research is surprising because today's Multiracial youth demographic (aged 0–18 years) is the fastest-growing racial group and the adult population has increased by 276% from 2010 to 2020, representing 10% of the US population.[1] Of the extant research, Multiracial youth compared with monoracial youth report lower levels of social belonging and various adverse mental health outcomes,[2,3] marking a need for pediatric health professionals to consider Multiracial identities.

This chapter discusses the impact of monoracial ideological, political, and clinical practices on medical research about Multiracial youth. Additionally, this chapter reviews challenges that monoracism[4] presents to Multiracial people, such as interpersonal/intergroup and systemic/institutional barriers and provides recommendations for pediatric health professionals to mitigate harm stemming from these experiences.

Defining Multiracial Identities

One of the biggest challenges that Multiracial people may face in health care, and other institutional settings, is the recognition and validation of their Multiracial identities. These challenges stem in part from historical complications with documentation of Multiracial identities. Although Multiracial people have existed throughout history, socially constructed racial classification systems have often masked recognition of the Multiracial group, enforcing the ideology of a singular racial group membership. In addition, historical legal policies in the United States also enforced the monoracial categorization of Multiracial people. Examples of these policies include the one-drop rule (ie, hypodescent), which enforced the categorization of a person with any Black or African American ancestry, regardless of other racial ancestry, as *Black* to reinforce oppressive societal hierarchies and the blood-quantum federal mandates, which limited Native American tribal citizenship. Thus, recognition of Multiracial people challenges the current racial classification system because Multiracial identity directly opposes essentialized historical and contemporary methods of determining racial and ethnic identities. With modern changes in demographic-enumeration practices used by the US Census Bureau (ie, its allowing for > 1 racial group selection) and increases in interracial marriages, recognition of the US Multiracial population has grown.

Multiracial Identity Challenges

Exclusion and Racial Ambiguity

As Multiracial people straddle boundaries between recognized monoracial groups, they are often perceived as marginal members of these groups. They do not easily fit into existing monoracial categories, a challenge resulting in higher rates of exclusion than monoracial groups experience.[5] Multiracial individuals may experience rejection, identity denial, and identity questioning (ie, "What are you?") from their multiple monoracial in-groups (eg, monoracial groups that their parents or caregivers belong to), which is often both psychologically and physically stressful.[6]

Pediatric health professionals should avoid reinforcing these experiences of identity denial for Multiracial patients. Still, challenges during patient-professional interactions may occur because of existing expectations about racial appearance. For example, Multiracial people may or may not physically match racial expectations for monoracial groups or they may appear racially ambiguous, creating uncertainty regarding their heritages. Notably, a Multiracial person may have a lighter or darker skin tone, but skin tone alone does not predict racial identification for Multiracial people.[7] Health professionals should not assume a Multiracial person's racial identification solely on the basis of the patient's skin tone. This advice extends to other identifiers such as names and language usage.[8]

Variability in racial appearance among the Multiracial population also suggests disparities in health outcomes based on perceived racial group membership. Among Multiracial people, those who are perceived by others as white, despite not identifying as white themselves, report better health status than Multiracial people who are not perceived as white.[9] This reporting is in line with the research finding that racial appearance is associated with disparities in health care treatment, such as prescribed pain medication.[10] Moreover, the effect of perceived racial group membership on Multiracial health outcomes may be further nuanced because the categorization of Multiracial people may be influenced by various factors, such as the gender of the observer.[11] Thus, different people may categorize a Multiracial individual as belonging to different racial groups, suggesting that Multiracial patients may experience inconsistent medical treatment by different health professionals, depending on how each professional racially perceives them.

Identity Flexibility and Demographic Forms

Whereas monoracial individuals' racial identities may match their biological parents', Multiracial individuals have a more variable path to establishing and claiming racial group membership. Some Multiracial individuals may claim membership to all their monoracial in-groups (eg, Black and Asian), some may identify with only one of their monoracial in-groups, and some may dismiss monoracial labels entirely and identify as Multiracial.[7] Additionally, there is often flexibility in how Multiracial people choose to identify racially at different stages of their lives and in different contexts (eg, with monoracial labels vs with a Multiracial label).[12] This variability in racial identity has proven challenging to capture on standard demographic forms. Moreover, the single forced-choice options (eg, "Please select one racial group") on demographic forms are unduly stressful for Multiracial people because they lead to decreased self-esteem, decreased motivation, increased anxiety, and lower belonging.[13,14]

Pediatric health professionals should be aware of these challenges in measuring racial identity. Forcing Multiracial-identified individuals into monoracial categories (eg, categorizing a patient as Black rather than Biracial Black/white) can also obscure patterns and increase errors in documenting health disparities between racial and ethnic groups.[15,16] This practice of racial categorization has contributed to a lack of knowledge surrounding health outcomes for Multiracial individuals. For example, Multiracial people may experience health disparities because of primary or secondary identification with different racial and ethnic in-groups.[17] Thus, an inclusive approach to demographic forms may both aid direction of needed research on this population and support development of Multiracial youth by validating identity challenges and shifts that children and adolescents experience.

Ongoing Challenges to Multiracial Youth Health Outcomes and Future Questions

It is important to avoid collapsing all Multiracial identities into one because they should not be treated as a monolith, especially when considering health disparities. Moreover, apart from other minority youth, Multiracial youth also experience Multiracial-specific challenges, such as higher health risks (eg, headaches, aches/pains, depression) and higher behavior risks (eg, substance use),[18] which persist across several Multiracial subgroups (eg, white/Black, white/Asian, Black/Native American). Thus, additional Multiracial health research is critical to provide tailored treatment and care for this growing demographic. For example, do Biracial Black/white people experience the same risk for hypertension, diabetes, and maternal death as monoracial Black adults? Do Multiracial Latino/a/e[a] people show the same "Hispanic health paradox"? Do Multiracial Asian people experience the same low access to health care as monoracial Asian American people? Finally, pediatric health professionals must become educated on known Multiracial health disparities, because racial and ethnic background affects clinical care issues, such as bone marrow donor matching. Multiracial patients experience significantly lower rates of finding donor matches, given that 85% of donors are white.[19]

---

[a] In this chapter, we use *Latino/a/e* when referring to people of Latin American origin or descent as a whole. It is a gender-neutral and gender-inclusive alternative to *Latino*. For a brief history of this term, including a rationale, refer to the book introduction.

Summary

Pediatric health professionals are responsible for validating, acknowledging, and reporting Multiracial backgrounds accurately and effectively. We also need to change and update our existing health disparities knowledge. Failure to change our practices, including of the demographic forms we use, the discussions we initiate, and the affirmations we make concerning a patient's racial identity will undermine the quality of professional-patient interactions. Further, Multiracial medical care will continue to follow a mythological and archaic monoracial framework, which will negatively serve this forever present and growing demographic.

Recommendations

Patient- and Family-Directed

- Make available inclusive demographic forms that allow for the selection of multiple racial options (eg, "Select all that apply") because this is vital for clarifying health-related research for all racial groups.

- Given that children can express racial and ethnic identities as early as 5 years old,[20] we suggest allowing children and adolescents to racially identify themselves on forms, or verbally, in addition to requesting demographic information from parents/caregivers.

- Provide each child and adolescent the opportunity to indicate their degree of identification with their selected racial and ethnic identities.[17]

- Allow children, adolescents, and parents/caregivers to complete demographic forms before each visit or periodically over time. This workflow may aid accommodation of identity flexibility and may change and create a more inclusive space for identity explorations, which are key to positive self-identification.

Clinical Practice/Organizations/Systems

- Pediatric health professionals should be cautious against assuming race and ethnicity on the basis of features such as skin tone and hair texture. Professionals should instead refer to either patient- or parent/caregiver-completed demographic forms, or verbal identification, over their own perceptions of the patient's (or parent's/caregiver's) racial and ethnic presentation. This approach will prevent miscategorization and identity denial for a Multiracial patient.

- Professionals should be cautious about assuming who is, or is not, a child's or adolescent's biological parent because parents may not always share physical characteristics with their children (eg, there may be varying skin tones).

- Professionals should encourage open discussion about racial and ethnic identities and cultural heritages with patients and parents/caregivers. Having one's Multiracial identity validated in a health care setting would show institutional support of that identity and the support of identity malleability.

● When Multiracial children and adolescents express their racial and ethnic identification, professionals, as well as parents and caregivers, should take care to avoid challenging or denying the specified racial identity (eg, "You're not *really* Black," "But you don't look Asian"). Rather, affirming one's Multiracial identity may protect against anxiety and depressive symptoms.[21]

References

1. Jones N, Marks R, Ramirez R, Rios-Vargas M. *2020 Census Illuminates Racial and Ethnic Composition of the Country.* US Census Bureau; 2021. Accessed March 13, 2023. https://www.census.gov/library/stories/2021/08/improved-race-ethnicity-measures-reveal-united-states-population-much-more-multiracial.html

2. Flores G, Lin H. Trends in racial/ethnic disparities in medical and oral health, access to care, and use of services in US children: has anything changed over the years? *Int J Equity Health.* 2013;12(1):10 PMID: 23339566 doi: 10.1186/1475-9276-12-10

3. Lau M, Lin H, Flores G. Racial/ethnic disparities in health and health care among U.S. adolescents. *Health Serv Res.* 2012;47(5):2031–2059 PMID: 22417169 doi: 10.1111/j.1475-6773.2012.01394.x

4. Johnston MP, Nadal KL. Multiracial microaggressions: exposing monoracism in everyday life and clinical practice. In: Sue DW, ed. *Microaggressions and Marginality: Manifestation, Dynamic, and Impact.* John Wiley & Sons Inc; 2010:123–145

5. Shih M, Sanchez DT. Perspectives and research on the positive and negative implications of having multiple racial identities. *Psychol Bull.* 2005;131(4):569–591 PMID: 16060803 doi: 10.1037/0033-2909.131.4.569

6. Albuja AF, Gaither SE, Sanchez DT, Straka B, Cipollina R. Psychophysiological stress responses to bicultural and Biracial identity denial. *J Soc Issues.* 2019;75(4):1165–1191 doi: 10.1111/josi.12347

7. Rockquemore KA, Brunsma DL, Delgado DJ. Racing to theory or retheorizing race? understanding the struggle to build a Multiracial identity theory. *J Soc Issues.* 2009;65(1):13–34 doi: 10.1111/j.1540-4560.2008.01585.x

8. Tsai A, Straka B, Gaither S. Mixed-heritage individuals' encounters with raciolinguistic ideologies. *J Multilingual Multicult Dev.* 2021:1–15 doi: 10.1080/01434632.2021.1904964

9. Jones CP, Truman BI, Elam-Evans LD, et al. Using "socially assigned race" to probe white advantages in health status. *Ethn Dis.* 2008;18(4):496–504 PMID: 19157256

10. Hoffman KM, Trawalter S, Axt JR, Oliver MN. Racial bias in pain assessment and treatment recommendations, and false beliefs about biological differences between blacks and whites. *Proc Natl Acad Sci U S A.* 2016;113(16):4296–4301 PMID: 27044069 doi: 10.1073/pnas.1516047113

11. Feliciano C. Shades of race: how phenotype and observer characteristics shape racial classification. *Am Behav Sci.* 2016;60(4):390–419 doi: 10.1177/0002764215613401

12. Harris DR, Sim JJ. Who is Multiracial? assessing the complexity of lived race. *Am Sociol Rev.* 2002;67(4):614–627 doi: 10.2307/3088948

13. Sanchez DT. How do forced-choice dilemmas affect Multiracial people? the role of identity autonomy and public regard in depressive symptoms. *J Appl Soc Psychol.* 2010;40(7):1657–1677 doi: 10.1111/j.1559-1816.2010.00634.x

14. Townsend SSM, Markus HR, Bergsieker HB. My choice, your categories: the denial of Multiracial identities. *J Soc Issues.* 2009;65(1):185–204 doi: 10.1111/j.1540-4560.2008.01594.x

15. Bratter JL, Gorman BK. Does Multiracial matter? a study of racial disparities in self-rated health. *Demography.* 2011;48(1):127–152 PMID: 21347806 doi: 10.1007/s13524-010-0005-0

16. Woolverton GA, Marks AK. "I just check 'other'": evidence to support expanding the measurement inclusivity and equity of ethnicity/race and cultural identifications of U.S. adolescents. *Cultur Divers Ethnic Minor Psychol.* 2023;29(1):64–73 PMID: 34351178 doi: 10.1037/cdp0000360

17. Wey A, Davis J, Juarez DT, Sentell T. Distinguishing between primary and secondary racial identification in analyses of health disparities of a Multiracial population in Hawaii. *Ethn Health.* 2018;23(3):233–248 PMID: 27905209 doi: 10.1080/13557858.2016.1263284

18. Udry JR, Li RM, Hendrickson-Smith J. Health and behavior risks of adolescents with mixed-race identity. *Am J Public Health.* 2003;93(11):1865–1870 PMID: 14600054 doi: 10.2105/AJPH.93.11.1865

19. Bergstrom TC, Garratt R, Sheehan-Connor D. Stem cell donor matching for patients of mixed race. *BE J Econ Anal Policy.* 2012;12(1): doi: 10.1515/1935-1682.3275

20. Ruble DN, Alvarez J, Bachman M, Cameron J. The development of a sense of "we": the emergence and implications of children's collective identity. In: Bennett M, Sani F, eds. *The Development of the Social Self.* Psychology Press; 2003:chap 2

21. Remedios JD, Chasteen AL. Finally, someone who "gets" me! Multiracial people value others' accuracy about their race. *Cultur Divers Ethnic Minor Psychol.* 2013;19(4):453–460 PMID: 23647325 doi: 10.1037/a0032249

Treaties, Public Health Service, and Health Status of Native American Children, Adolescents, and Young Adults

Joseph Burns, MD, and Allison Empey, MD (Confederated Tribes of Grand Ronde)

Children learn from what they see. We need to set an example of truth and action.

Howard Rainer, Taos Pueblo-Creek

Foundations of Inequity

Since first European contact, Native American populations have experienced inequities in health.[1,2] Although the evidence lags because of underreporting or misclassification of race and ethnicity data, there are egregious inequities in American Indian/Alaska Native (AI/AN) child health reports relative to the general population. These health inequities are driven by historical and current systemic racism.

People of AI/AN heritage have experienced significant historical trauma, described as a succession of intergenerational emotional and psychological injury.[3] Since first settler contact, colonization has aimed to erase AI/AN communities through the loss of land, language, spiritual practices, and culture.[3] Historically, federal legislation, through systemically racist policies such as Indian boarding schools, forced relocations, and land allocation, and currently, the chronic underfunding of the Indian Health Service (IHS), continues to support these aims, predisposing communities to trauma, stress, and illness.[4]

The US government contributed to deliberate ethnocide through the Indian boarding school system. From the 1860s through as late as the 1960s, Native American children were forcibly removed from their homes and communities, losing connection to their cultures, families, and nations. These institutions aimed to eliminate Indigenous identities through forced assimilation in dress, language, and culture. Among survivors, the boarding school system has been associated with high rates of physical, emotional, and sexual abuse leading to numerous health issues affecting generations to come.[5,6] Increased attention to this issue has manifested in a federal investigation into the federal Indian boarding schools to further substantiate the scope of abuse and the long-term consequences of 150 years of the boarding school system on AI/AN populations.[6]

Relocation through federal policy has dramatically affected AI/AN populations. Numerous forced removals, including the Indian Removal Act of 1830, which permitted the Trail of Tears, displaced millions of AI/AN people. These deliberate attempts to infringe on

Indigenous sovereignty persisted into the 20th century, with the Indian Relocation Act of 1956, which aimed to shift AI/AN populations to urban centers, further severing ties to Indigenous lands and practices. This upheaval and lack of sense of place and belonging has contributed significantly to historical trauma in AI/AN populations.[4]

These ordeals result in exposure to adverse childhood experiences (ACEs), including psychological and physical abuse, violence, or substance use, manifesting in an intergenerational and epigenetic predisposition to poor health outcomes.[7] In addition, increasing ACEs are associated with smoking, obesity, depression, suicidality, substance use, cancer, cardiovascular disease, and sexually transmitted infections.[7]

Continued Intergenerational Impacts

Historical trauma continues to affect children, adolescents, and families today. Children and adolescents from AI/AN populations experience health inequities, including higher rates of obesity, type 2 diabetes, cardiovascular disease, substance use, and suicide than the general population.[1] The COVID-19 pandemic and a disproportionate number of cases and deaths of AI/AN people compared with the general population cast new light on the factors driving health inequities in AI/AN communities, including past and current policies that have kept AI/AN people in poverty and without access to high-quality, culturally relevant health care.[8] These factors include limited school funding, which is largely driven by property tax; federal redlining, which limited access to home ownership; and predatory loans, to name a few.[2]

American Indian/Alaska Native children, adolescents, and young adults are affected by obesity at far higher rates and earlier in life than the general population.[9] Obesity is associated with hypertension, insulin resistance, and premature death.[10] In one of the largest longitudinal cohorts following AI/AN adolescents, 24.9% met the criteria for the diagnosis of metabolic syndrome.[9] These factors are driven by social determinants of health, including the built environment, such as limited availability of parks and green spaces and proximity to highways and industrial spaces, lack of access to healthful foods, lack of opportunities for exercise, poor air quality, and heavy metal exposure, many of which result from systemically racist policies based on land allocation, infrastructure design, and waste management.[2,9]

The age-adjusted suicide rate for AI/AN children and adolescents is 3 to 6 times higher than for the general population.[1] It represents the second-leading cause of death for AI/AN youth between 10 and 24 years of age.[11] The risk for suicide is associated with increased ACEs, with evidence suggesting increased rates of these factors for AI/AN communities because of rampant historical trauma and settler colonialism.[1,11] Refer to Chapter 12, Addressing the Impact of Racism on the Mental Health of Youth: A Focus on Pediatric Health Professionals and Collaborators.

Substance use is more common among AI/AN adolescents in AI/AN populations than in other demographics, with 18.3% of adolescents between the ages of 14 and 16 years meeting the diagnostic criteria for substance use disorders.[1] A recent study evaluating substance use disorder in AI/AN adults showed that both historical trauma secondary to colonialism and persistent microaggressive behaviors toward AI/AN populations contribute to suboptimal behavioral health.[12] Discrimination and bias also affect access to treatment.[12] Acknowledging racial trauma in treatment and adequately addressing the historical context of this inequity is also required for health professionals to address substance use in AI/AN communities.[12]

Inequity in Health Care, Education, and Income

The deliberate attempts to eliminate Indigenous peoples and practices through relocation, the Indian boarding school system, and ongoing threats embedded within settler colonialism have led to social determinants of health dictated by structural racism. The perceived superiority of the colonizing culture permits racist policies that continue to affect Indigenous child and adolescent health outcomes. Despite ample evidence supporting the increased risk for adverse effects, many policies and cultural practices still exist today, including inadequate funding for the IHS, lack of representation of AI/AN in government and society, and constant attacks on Native nation sovereignty.

The IHS is woefully underfunded. For members of federally recognized Native nations, care may be obtained through the IHS, Native nation health organizations, or Urban Indian Health Centers. However, the funding for each of these sources varies widely. Native nation–operated health facilities may have more control over funding allocation and an improved understanding of community needs but may face challenges acquiring health care funds.[13] Additionally, many nation members live in urban cities or far from their nation health facilities because of relocations, making access difficult. Recruitment and retention of health professionals is a persistent challenge for the IHS. Staffing of these sites is often inadequate, with IHS vacancy rates for all health professions at 25%.[14] Native American people experience discrimination and interpersonal racism in the health care setting. In one study, more than 20% of the 342 participants self-identifying as AI/AN reported discrimination in a clinical encounter and 15% avoided seeking care because of anticipated discrimination.[15] Refer to Chapter 3, Implicit and Explicit Biases and the Pediatric Health Professional.

The educational attainment rate for AI/AN populations is the lowest of any demographic in the United States.[16] American Indian/Alaska Native students contend that traditional American curricula fail to engage with AI/AN students in meaningful ways, often being deemed culturally irrelevant by the learners themselves.[16] The deliberate exclusion of AI/AN history and culture from mainstream curricula is yet another colonial aggression, furthering the historical trauma experienced by these populations.[16] Limited educational attainment likely dramatically affects health literacy, hindering the ability to obtain and comprehend information critical to adherence to health-related planning and guidance. In addition, under-enrollment in college and medical education furthers the underrepresentation of AI/AN populations in the health professions.[17]

Finally, the shortage of AI/AN health professionals limits the ability of professionals to shape workforce culture, culturally connect in meaningful ways with AI/AN patients, build relationships with Native nation leadership, and foster a community of strength- and resilience-based medicine. Ongoing efforts dedicated to improving exposure to STEM disciplines in a culturally relevant manner may improve AI/AN educational attainment and representation in the health professions.[17]

More than 25% of AI/AN populations experience poverty, a rate more than double the general population's.[1] This rate is even higher for AI/AN children, with 32% for families with children younger than 5 years.[1] In addition, the unemployment rate is as high as 35%, driven by a lack of economic development and the geographic isolation in AI/AN lands secondary to relocation, which lends to low-wage jobs.[1] Continued efforts to improve education and to broaden opportunities in a more diverse workforce will improve these rates and overall AI/AN child health.

Summary

Pediatric health professionals, allied health professionals, and community partners play an essential role in helping identify children at risk for health inequities and in advocating for policies combating structural racism.

Recommendations

Patient- and Family-Directed

- Take a strength-based approach that acknowledges Indigenous families' and patients' cultural strength and resilience.[11]
- It is essential to be aware of AI/AN resources in the communities to partner with local Indigenous entities. This partnership will allow pediatric health professionals to understand the priorities, needs, and historical experiences of local Indigenous populations and leverage their cultural assets and resilience to preserve Indigenous identities and overall health.

Clinical Practice/Organizations/Systems

- In clinical and hospital settings, pediatric health professionals can use trauma-informed, culturally relevant screening tools to screen for ACEs, social determinants of health, and sexual trafficking.[11] These include resources available through the American Academy of Pediatrics Trauma Toolbox for Primary Care.[18]
- To maximize effectiveness, pediatric health professionals should use culturally relevant messaging toward AI/AN populations. Recently, efforts to improve COVID-19 vaccination rates have included content about protecting culture, language, and elders. As an example, innovative vaccination initiatives include immunizing elders to serve as role models for others and prioritizing community outreach for those unable to travel to vaccination clinics.[19]

- Implement trauma-informed care in clinical settings. Several evidence-based interventions have been designed to meet the specific needs of AI/AN children to mitigate the consequences of historical trauma, settler colonialism, and racism. Among these are trauma-informed treatment guides from the National Native Children's Trauma Center and anti-racism resources from the American Academy of Pediatrics and state chapters.[20,21]

- Support efforts to improve exposure to STEM disciplines among AI/AN children, adolescents, and young adults to cultivate a workforce that reflects AI/AN populations sharing geography with the United States. Although several pathway programs exist to support AI/AN physicians, the training, recruiting, and retaining of talented AI/AN pediatricians serving IHS, Native nation, and Urban Indian care facilities is critical.

Public Health Policy and Community Advocacy

- At the advocacy level, pediatric health professionals and organizations can advocate for increased funding for the IHS and continued respect for Native nation sovereignty. Respecting nation sovereignty requires understanding that nations have the right to self-govern their people and territories and to self-determine their futures.

References

1. Sarche M, Spicer P. Poverty and health disparities for American Indian and Alaska Native children: current knowledge and future prospects. *Ann N Y Acad Sci*. 2008;1136(1):126–136 PMID: 18579879 doi: 10.1196/annals.1425.017

2. Empey A, Garcia A, Bell S. American Indian/Alaska Native child health and poverty. *Acad Pediatr*. 2021;21(8S)(suppl):S134–S139 PMID: 34740420 doi: 10.1016/j.acap.2021.07.026

3. Brave Heart MYH. The historical trauma response among natives and its relationship with substance abuse: a Lakota illustration. *J Psychoactive Drugs*. 2003;35(1):7–13 PMID: 12733753 doi: 10.1080/02791072.2003.10399988

4. Burns J, Angelino AC, Lewis K, et al. Land rights and health outcomes in American Indian/Alaska Native children. *Pediatrics*. 2021;148(5):e2020041350 PMID: 34706902 doi: 10.1542/peds.2020-041350

5. Running Bear U, Thayer ZM, Croy CD, Kaufman CE, Manson SM; AI-SUPERPFP Team. The impact of individual and parental American Indian boarding school attendance on chronic physical health of Northern Plains Tribes. *Fam Community Health*. 2019;42(1):1–7 PMID: 30431464 doi: 10.1097/FCH.0000000000000205

6. Newland B; Indian Affairs. *Federal Indian Boarding School Initiative Investigative Report*. US Dept of the Interior; 2022:1–106

7. Warne D, Dulacki K, Spurlock M, et al. Adverse childhood experiences (ACE) among American Indians in South Dakota and associations with mental health conditions, alcohol use, and smoking. *J Health Care Poor Underserved*. 2017;28(4):1559–1577 PMID: 29176114 doi: 10.1353/hpu.2017.0133

8. Burki T. COVID-19 among American Indians and Alaska Natives. *Lancet Infect Dis*. 2021;21(3):325–326 PMID: 33639126 doi: 10.1016/S1473-3099(21)00083-9

9. Deen JF, Adams AK, Fretts A, et al. Cardiovascular disease in American Indian and Alaska Native youth: unique risk factors and areas of scholarly need. *J Am Heart Assoc*. 2017;6(10):e007576 PMID: 29066451 doi: 10.1161/JAHA.117.007576

10. Franks PW, Hanson RL, Knowler WC, Sievers ML, Bennett PH, Looker HC. Childhood obesity, other cardiovascular risk factors, and premature death. *N Engl J Med*. 2010;362(6):485–493 PMID: 20147714 doi: 10.1056/NEJMoa0904130

11. Bell S, Deen JF, Fuentes M, Moore K; American Academy of Pediatrics Committee on Native American Child Health. Caring for American Indian and Alaska Native children and adolescents. *Pediatrics*. 2021;147(4):e2021050498 PMID: 33753539 doi: 10.1542/peds.2021-050498

12. Skewes MC, Blume AW. Understanding the link between racial trauma and substance use among American Indians. *Am Psychol*. 2019;74(1):88–100 PMID: 30652902 doi: 10.1037/amp0000331

13. Warne D, Frizzell LB. American Indian health policy: historical trends and contemporary issues. *Am J Public Health*. 2014;104(suppl 3):S263–S267 PMID: 24754649 doi: 10.2105/AJPH.2013.301682

14. Government Accountability Office. *Indian Health Service: Agency Faces Ongoing Challenges Filling Provider Vacancies*. Government Accountability Office; 2018. Accessed February 1, 2023. https://www.gao.gov/assets/gao-18-580-highlights.pdf

15. Findling MG, Casey LS, Fryberg SA, et al. Discrimination in the United States: experiences of Native Americans. *Health Serv Res*. 2019;54(suppl 2):1431–1441 PMID: 31657013 doi: 10.1111/1475-6773.13224

16. Martinez D. School culture and American Indian educational outcome. *Procedia Soc Behav Sci*. 2014;116:199–205 doi: 10.1016/j.sbspro.2014.01.194

17. Persaud D, Burns J. First Nations People: addressing the relationships between under-enrollment in medical education, STEM education, and health in the United States. *Societies (Basel)*. 2018;8(1):9 doi: 10.3390/soc8010009

18. American Academy of Pediatrics. Supporting children who have experienced trauma. Foster Care. Accessed March 13, 2023. https://www.aap.org/en/patient-care/foster-care/supporting-children-who-have-experienced-trauma/#traumatoolbox

19. Foxworth R, Redvers N, Moreno MA, Lopez-Carmen VA, Sanchez GR, Shultz JM. COVID-19 vaccination in American Indians and Alaska Natives—lessons from effective community responses. *N Engl J Med*. 2021;385(26):2403–2406 PMID: 34919356 doi: 10.1056/NEJMp2113296

20. Administration for Children & Families. Resources specific to American Indian/Alaskan Native (AI/AN) communities. Resource Guide to Trauma-Informed Human Services. Accessed February 1, 2023. https://www.acf.hhs.gov/trauma-toolkit/american-indian-alaskan-native-communities

21. Bright Futures. Health equity resources for health care professionals. Bright Futures in Clinical Practice. Accessed March 13, 2023. https://www.aap.org/en/practice-management/bright-futures/bright-futures-in-clinical-practice/bright-futures-health-equity-resources-for-health-care-professionals

CHAPTER 8

The Model Minority Myth

Y. Joel Wong, PhD, and Jonathan Kang, MS

Introduction to the Model Minority Myth

The model minority myth (MMM) is a cluster of oppressive ideologies and stereotypes that frame certain racially minoritized groups in the United States, especially Asian Americans, as more successful and hardworking than other minoritized groups that may be depicted as being lazy or having inappropriate cultural values.[1] The historical roots of the MMM can be traced to a 1966 article by the sociologist William Petersen, who described Japanese Americans as successful because of their hard work, respect for authority, and self-reliance.[2] Over time, this stereotype has been generalized to other Asian American ethnic groups and to other non-Asian minoritized groups, such as Black Caribbean and African immigrants.[3,4] This chapter examines the dimensions and consequences of the MMM, critiques its validity, and elucidates its implications in pediatric health care. We primarily focus on Asian Americans while acknowledging that the *model minority myth*, as a term, has also been applied to other minoritized groups.

Dimensions of the MMM

The MMM consists of a cluster of overlapping ideas that are both stereotypical (generalizations of racially minoritized groups) and ideological (prescriptions of what racially minoritized groups should do).[1] First, the myth depicts Asian Americans as both universally intelligent and academically and occupationally successful. This success is attributed to Asian Americans' cultural values, such as hard work and filial piety.[5] Second, Asian Americans are portrayed as having few academic or health challenges, so they seem to face few barriers to success.[5] A broader implication of the MMM is that other Americans may not even perceive Asian Americans as racially minoritized groups in need of resources accorded to other minoritized groups.[6] Perhaps the most insidious dimension of the MMM is that it oppresses other racially minoritized groups by putting Asian Americans and Black immigrants, given their so-called success through hard work, in opposition to other minoritized groups, such as US-born Black Americans, who are often inaccurately and unfairly accused of lacking a positive work ethic, despite being subject to intergenerational effects of persistent, legalized racism.[1] Consequently, the MMM should be challenged as a racist ideology that oppresses all communities of color, not just Asian Americans, by buttressing the myth of meritocracy, or the idea that any group can succeed solely through hard work.[7]

Challenging the Validity of the MMM

The validity of the MMM has been contested on several grounds by scholars. It is undermined by research that indicates inequalities among groups identified within the MMM. Disaggregation of data about Asian Americans, a disparate group comprising more than 20 ethnic groups, has uncovered large within-group differences that rebut the MMM. First, although a higher percentage of Asian Americans (53.5%) have college degrees than the overall US population (31.5%), several Asian American ethnic groups, such as Hmong (19.8%), Cambodians (18.3%) and Laotians (16.6%), experience low rates of college degree attainment.[8] Second, children and adolescents of Southeast Asian immigrant parents experience higher rates of physical and mental health conditions than those from other Asian American demographic groups and white children born in the United States.[9] Third, 76% of Asian Americans, a percentage equivalent to that of Black Americans, reported that they experience race-based discrimination, with Asian Americans having been particularly discriminated against during the COVID-19 pandemic through racial scapegoating.[10,11(p19)]

Negative Consequences of the MMM

Although the MMM comprises seemingly positive stereotypes, it has many harmful consequences. Any stereotypes that disregard an individual's unique personhood cause psychological distress. For example, Asian American college students who were told that their race implied traits associated with the MMM (eg, good at math, hardworking, ambitious) reported greater feelings of anger and frustration caused by depersonalization.[12] Beyond creating the distress of denied individuality, positive stereotypes come paired with negative implications. For instance, although the MMM portrays Asian Americans as smart, hardworking, and successful, it is inextricably tied to unfavorable stereotypes, such as meekness, social ineptitude, and physical weakness.[13] The awareness that positive stereotypes reflect prejudice is not lost on individuals who have been racially marginalized, causing further distress to the individuals when subjected to the stereotypes.[14] Subjugation by the MMM also leads to further harm by engendering interracial resentment and discrimination caused by positive biases that seemingly favor Asian American youth. For example, the bullying of Asian American students in school may result from teachers favoring Asian American students.[15,16]

Because of the prescriptive nature of the MMM, many Asian American youth may internalize the assumption that they must be academically successful, which can lead to chronic stress and self-doubt when these high standards are not met.[5] Further, the pressure of the MMM has been linked to a lack of help-seeking behaviors, such that non-Hispanic Asian adolescents were the least likely to seek out school mental health services (5,972 out of 165,686 participants), according to a study that used public-use data from the 2009 to 2019 National Survey on Drug Use and Health.[17] This link reinforces perceptions that Asian American youth are less vulnerable to mental health issues, and a vicious cycle is perpetuated that limits their access to and use of support resources (eg, community organizations and mental health services) relative to other racially minoritized groups, despite urgent need. In these ways, internalized expectations of the MMM may be associated with increased risk for and prevalence of unaddressed mental health conditions.

Practical Implications for Pediatric Health Professionals

Several implications for pediatric health professionals and other adolescent- and young adult–serving professionals can be gleaned from the following review. Unfortunately, the pervasiveness of the MMM has led to a lack of Asian American and Black immigrant health-related research and to lower coverage, access, and quality of health care, thus contributing to the invisibility of their health needs.[18] Therefore, the most vital practical implication is for pediatric health professionals to advocate for greater funding, resources, and policies that can benefit Asian Americans and Black immigrants subjugated by the MMM. Advocacy may also involve collecting and reporting disaggregated health data on diverse ethnic and immigrant groups to uncover which subgroups experience higher risk for adverse health outcomes.[19] Health professionals are also encouraged to raise awareness of the inaccuracy of the MMM and its negative effects on minoritized groups.

We encourage pediatric health professionals to attend training programs on the MMM. Indeed, evidence from experimental research suggests that the MMM can trigger the perception that Asian Americans experience better mental health and fewer clinical symptoms, which can lead to overlooking resources and referrals for care for patients.[20] Pediatric health professionals can be trained to be vigilant against MMM biases in health care decisions by implementing 3 evidence-based anti-stereotypical strategies: counter-stereotypical exemplars, implementation intentions, and structured free recalls. Exposure to counter-stereotypical exemplars of an ethnic group (eg, stories of Asian Americans who have health concerns) might help mitigate the influence of the MMM in health care decisions.[21] This strategy can be paired with implementation intentions, which translate health professionals' consciously held equitable values into automatically triggered cognitions and actions that inhibit implicit model minority stereotypes through if-then reminders (eg, "If I spend time with an Asian American patient, then I will remind myself of stories of Asian Americans with diverse health needs).[22] Unfortunately, this strategy may apply less to Black immigrant groups because of the link between health status and one's ability to immigrate to the United States and the stigmatization that results from group affiliation to a disease process (refer to Chapter 10, The Intersection of Racism, Immigration, and Child Health).

Another strategy is structured free recalls that reduce health professionals' reliance on the overall evaluation of a patient's health, which could be biased by the MMM.[23] For instance, pediatric health professionals could note evidence for and against a diagnosis or treatment on the basis of predetermined medical guidelines rather than allow implicit biases to dominate medical decision-making.

Summary

The MMM is a cluster of racist ideologies that depict Asian Americans, and, to some extent, Black immigrants, as smart and hardworking people who lack impediments to success and experience more success than the other US racially minoritized groups. Pediatric health professionals are encouraged to actively resist the influence of the MMM on health care practices and policies.

Recommendations

Patient- and Family-Directed

- Expose yourself to counter-stereotypical exemplars of Asian Americans and Black immigrants to mitigate the influence of the MMM on health care decisions.
- Use implementation intentions (if-then reminders) to prevent applying model minority stereotypes to patients.
- To guard against applying stereotypes to patients based on the MMM, note evidence for and against a diagnosis or treatment decision on the basis of predetermined medical guidelines.

Clinical Practice/Organizations/Systems

- Attend training programs to challenge the MMM.

Public Health Policy and Community Advocacy

- Advocate for greater funding, resources, and policies that benefit groups subjugated by the MMM, while being careful not to undermine advances for youth from historically aggrieved groups still challenged by racism, such as Black American descendants of enslaved people and Native Americans/Alaska Natives.
- Disaggregate health data on diverse Asian American, Black immigrant, and other minoritized groups that can uncover which subgroups experience higher risk for adverse health outcomes.

References

1. Yi V, Mac J, Na VS, et al. Toward an anti-imperialistic critical race analysis of the model minority myth. *Rev Educ Res.* 2020;90(4):542–579 doi: 10.3102/0034654320933532
2. Pettersen W. Success story, Japanese-American style. *New York Times.* January 9, 1966. Accessed February 2, 2023. https://www.nytimes.com/1966/01/09/archives/success-story-japaneseamerican-style-success-story-japaneseamerican.html
3. Ukpokodu ON. African immigrants, the "new model minority": examining the reality in U.S. k-12 schools. *Urban Rev.* 2018;50(1):69–96 doi: 10.1007/s11256-017-0430-0
4. Ifatunji MA. A test of the Afro Caribbean model minority hypothesis: exploring the role of cultural attributes in labor market disparities between African Americans and Afro Caribbeans. *Du Bois Rev.* 2016;13(1):109–138 doi: 10.1017/S1742058X16000035

5. Yoo HC, Burrola KS, Steger MF. A preliminary report on a new measure: internalization of the Model Minority Myth Measure (IM-4) and its psychological correlates among Asian American college students. *J Couns Psychol*. 2010;57(1):114–127 PMID: 21133563 doi: 10.1037/a0017871

6. Museus SD, Kiang PN. Deconstructing the model minority myth and how it contributes to the invisible minority reality in higher education research. *New Dir Institutional Res*. 2009;2009(142):5–15 doi: 10.1002/ir.292

7. Poon O, Squire D, Kodama C, et al. A critical review of the model minority myth in selected literature on Asian Americans and Pacific Islanders in higher education. *Rev Educ Res*. 2016;86(2):469–502 doi: 10.3102/0034654315612205

8. Community facts. AAPI Data. Accessed February 2, 2023. http://facts.aapidata.com/nationaldata

9. Huang KY, Calzada E, Cheng S, Brotman LM. Physical and mental health disparities among young children of Asian immigrants. *J Pediatr*. 2012;160(2):331–336.e1 PMID: 21907351 doi: 10.1016/j.jpeds.2011.08.005

10. Horowitz JM, Brown A, Cox K. Race in America 2019. Pew Research Center. April 9, 2019. Accessed February 2, 2023. https://www.pewresearch.org/social-trends/2019/04/09/race-in-america-2019

11. Cheng HL, Wong YJ, Li PFJ, McDermott RC. COVID-19 racism, anxiety, and racial/ethnic attitudes among Asian American college students. *Couns Psychol Q*. 2022;35(4):897–920 doi: 10.1080/09515070.2021.1988514

12. Siy JO, Cheryan S. When compliments fail to flatter: American individualism and responses to positive stereotypes. *J Pers Soc Psychol*. 2013;104(1):87–102 PMID: 23025500 doi: 10.1037/a0030183

13. Lin MH, Kwan VSY, Cheung A, Fiske ST. Stereotype content model explains prejudice for an envied outgroup: scale of anti-Asian American stereotypes. *Pers Soc Psychol Bull*. 2005;31(1):34–47 PMID: 15574660 doi: 10.1177/0146167204271320

14. Siy JO, Cheryan S. Prejudice masquerading as praise: the negative echo of positive stereotypes. *Pers Soc Psychol Bull*. 2016;42(7):941–954 PMID: 27287753 doi: 10.1177/0146167216649605

15. Qin DB, Way N, Rana M. The "model minority" and their discontent: examining peer discrimination and harassment of Chinese American immigrant youth. *New Dir Child Adolesc Dev*. 2008;2008(121):27–42 PMID: 18792949 doi: 10.1002/cd.221

16. Liang B, Grossman JM, Deguchi M. Chinese American middle school youths' experiences of discrimination and stereotyping. *Qual Res Psychol*. 2007;4(1–2):187–205 doi: 10.1080/14780880701473599

17. Wilk AS, Hu JC, Wen H, Cummings JR. Recent trends in school-based mental health services among low-income and racial and ethnic minority adolescents. *JAMA Pediatr*. 2022;176(8):813–815 PMID: 35499844 doi: 10.1001/jamapediatrics.2022.1020

18. Jang D, Suraprui A. Not the model minority: how to address disparities in Asian American health care. *Asian Am Policy Rev*. 2009;18:91–106

19. Wong YJ, Vaughan EL, Liu T, Chang TK. Asian Americans' proportion of life in the United States and suicide ideation: the moderating effects of ethnic subgroups. *Asian Am J Psychol*. 2014;5(3):237–242 doi: 10.1037/a0033283

20. Cheng AW, Chang J, O'Brien J, Budgazad MS, Tsai J. Model minority stereotype: influence on perceived mental health needs of Asian Americans. *J Immigr Minor Health*. 2017;19(3):572–581 PMID: 27246287 doi: 10.1007/s10903-016-0440-0

21. FitzGerald C, Martin A, Berner D, Hurst S. Interventions designed to reduce implicit prejudices and implicit stereotypes in real world contexts: a systematic review. *BMC Psychol*. 2019;7(1):29 PMID: 31097028 doi: 10.1186/s40359-019-0299-7

22. Mendoza SA, Gollwitzer PM, Amodio DM. Reducing the expression of implicit stereotypes: reflexive control through implementation intentions. *Pers Soc Psychol Bull.* 2010;36(4):512–523 PMID: 20363905 doi: 10.1177/0146167210362789

23. Baltes BB, Bauer CB, Frensch PA. Does a structured free recall intervention reduce the effect of stereotypes on performance ratings and by what cognitive mechanism? *J Appl Psychol.* 2007;92(1):151–164 PMID: 17227157 doi: 10.1037/0021-9010.92.1.151

The Intersection of Race, Sexuality, and Gender Identity During Adolescence

Nadia Dowshen, MD, MSHP, and Renata Arrington Sanders, MD, MPH, ScM

"I feel like I'm different but not in a bad way. I feel like I'm just like me, like I live my life as—I live my life for me, so I feel like it's just me being me..."

—A 19-year-old Biracial gay-identified, cisgender man enrolled in the Providing Unique Support for Health (PUSH) Study describing their identity and the complexities of navigating multiple identities

Introduction

Adolescence, the transition period from childhood to adulthood, is a time for youth to gain independence and establish a secure identity. Progression occurs through cognitive, psychosocial, and emotional maturation, including advanced reasoning and abstract thinking, identity formation, and self-regulation.[1] An adolescent may formulate multiple social identities (eg, racial, ethnic, sexual, and gender) during adolescence. This confluence of identities is known as *intersectionality*. Racial or ethnic identity, for example, is based on a common heritage and a shared sense of identity, affecting one's internal self-concept and interactions with others.[2] Sexual identity involves 2 processes: *identity formation*, consisting of awareness, questioning, and exploration of one's sexuality, and *identity integration*, incorporation of sexuality into one's self-concept.[3] Identity integration for LGBTQ+ youth further includes involvement in more prominent lesbian, gay, bisexual, or other social activities oriented toward nonheterosexual sexual orientation groups; resolving homonegative attitudes; and becoming comfortable with others knowing about one's sexual identity and disclosing the identity to others. Developing one's gender identity can be a complicated process for some, whereas it can be marked by early permanence for others. Gender is a socially derived concept based on roles and societal expectations about behaviors, characteristics, and thoughts that typically go along with sex assigned at birth. Gender identity is a personally known and defined construct based on one's basic sense of being male, female, or another gender.[4] Transgender and gender-diverse identities, binary and nonbinary alike, may be asserted or expressed as early as the age of 4 or 5 years.

Identity Intersectionality and Minority Stress

Intersectionality is a theoretical framework suggesting that individuals have multiple social identities that intersect and increase their risk for disadvantage or discrimination because of the larger socio-structural inequities they experience.[5] Coined by Crenshaw,[5] the concept of intersectionality recognizes that people with overlapping identities may experience oppression and discrimination because of socio-structural inequities that are not simply additive but interdependent and mutually reinforcing.[6] For example, young Black gay and bisexual men may experience a conflict between same-sex sexuality and cultural expectations of masculinity and religious morality during critical moments in adolescent development.[7] In a group in which racial identity may be more significant to self-concept than sexual identity,[8] nondisclosure may be protective and adaptive by allowing these men to preserve critical social supports. However, adolescents feeling forced to hide their sexual orientation or same-sex sexual activity may experience significant isolation at a time when interpersonal attachments are essential for healthy development. This isolation may predispose some adolescents to engage in potentially riskier sexual activity that is secretive and unprotected.[9]

Disadvantage and discrimination may result from the marginalization and minority stress experienced within LGBTQ+ communities.[10] The theory of *minority stress* posits that individuals who identify as members of groups that have been stigmatized and minoritized, in this case, who identify as members of LGBTQ+ communities, or gender-diverse communities, experience discrimination and harassment because of their identities, which cause stress and trauma that may ultimately lead to adverse mental and physical health outcomes.[11,12] Stress and poor outcomes can occur because of experiences that relate to internalized homonegativity (ie, internalized negative views about identifying as gay), transphobia, stigma, and limited social connectedness. For example, transgender preadolescents and adolescents experience higher risk for suicidal ideation and suicide attempts. Still, it is important to be clear that this results from gender minority stress, shame, and stigma that they face from factors such as bullying and lack of parental acceptance, rather than being transgender.[13] On the other hand, parental support has been shown to promote resilience in gay and transgender adolescents, mitigate the impacts of minority stress, and decrease the risk for suicide.[14]

In adolescents with intersecting minoritized racial and ethnic identities, minority stress caused by sexual or gender identity is also compounded by racism.[15] LGBTQ+ adolescents and young adults who identify as Black, Indigenous, and People of Color (BIPOC) experience higher rates of emotional, physical, and sexual abuse; poorer mental health (eg, 35% of gender-expansive adolescents report a past suicide attempt); and reduced academic achievement than their heterosexual, cisgender peers.[16] Structural and interpersonal racism have decreased access to health care. LGBTQ+ adolescents who identify as BIPOC experience disproportionately higher rates of HIV than their white cisgender, heterosexual counterparts because of the effects of structural racism, including factors such as socioeconomic inequity, the built environment (eg, redlining and economic segregation), and mass incarceration.[16,17] Black and Latinx[a] sexual minority men and transgender women experience high levels of unstable housing because of discrimination related to their sexual orientation and gender identity. This displacement has been found to contribute to high rates of transactional sex and sexual risk, which contribute to high rates of sexually transmitted infection and HIV infection.[18]

Summary

Despite the prevalence of stigma, discrimination, and marginalization, most LGBTQ+ adolescents who identify as BIPOC demonstrate remarkable resilience, develop coping strategies, build social support networks, and experience good mental health. As a result, there has been a call for intersectional interventions to address gaps in mental health, sexual risk, and primary care.[7] Such interventions need to consider the interdependence of multiple co-occurring, devalued social identities in LGBTQ+ adolescents who identify as BIPOC and need to incorporate multilevel strategies to address discrimination specific to different identity groups and perceived and actual experiences of marginalization in school, community, and pediatric settings.[10] One first step is to enhance awareness of inequality and stigma (eg, critical consciousness, racial awareness) in adolescents and their pediatric health professionals, which has been shown to have long-term and protective effects on health and well-being.[19] Programs will need to promote strong prosocial identities among adolescents to mitigate the adverse health effects of discrimination and marginalization. In addition, understanding the components of intersecting identities (eg, racial centrality, religiosity and spirituality, and social support) can offer protection, foster resilience, and, sometimes, buffer the adverse effects existing within multiple identities that have been marginalized.

Recommendations

Patient- and Family-Directed

● Recognize that interventions or treatment plans for adolescents need to be *culturally congruent*, meaning that they consider an adolescent's intersecting identities.

● Include confidential time in all adolescent visits to ask about the adolescent's sexual and gender identities and how they intersect with other identities and experiences.

● Provide a safe and inclusive clinical environment that allows adolescents to feel comfortable with sharing and receiving support for their intersectional identities. For example, in reception areas, display Pride flags that include racial diversity and that celebrate different racial and ethnic groups. In addition, ensure that printed materials focusing on sexuality and gender identity also include racial diversity, as well as discuss the impacts of racism.

---

[a] In this chapter, we use *Latinx* when referring to people of Latin American origin or descent as a whole. It is a gender-neutral and gender-inclusive alternative to *Latino*. For a brief history of this term, including a rationale, refer to the book introduction.

Clinical Practice/Organizations/Systems

- Hire diverse staff with respect to racial and ethnic identities and sexual and gender identities because representation is critical for adolescents to receive the maximum care benefits.

- For all staff across disciplines, require diversity and inclusion and/or unconscious bias training that provides skills around caring for patients with intersectional identities and around the impacts of racism and heterosexism on the health and well-being of adolescents.

- Use trauma-informed practices, which are critical for all adolescents, especially those with intersecting racial and ethnic and sexual and gender minority identities because these adolescents are more likely to have experienced trauma in relation to their identities.

Public Health Policy and Community Advocacy

- Become familiar with local community resources that may support LGBTQ+ adolescents and their families with intersecting racial and ethnic minority identities.

- Refer to formal and informal community-based organizations that can provide social support, foster resilience, and create a community of connectedness. For example, local Pride centers, House Ball coalitions, school gender and sexuality alliances, PFLAG groups, Black- and Latinx-specific community-based organizations for HIV prevention, and places of worship can be resources for direct services or as a connection to services.

- Partner with local and state government and policy stakeholders to ensure supportive environments for gender and sexual minority adolescents with intersecting racial and ethnic minority identities in schools, health care settings, and other public spaces. For example, many pediatric health professionals have provided expert testimony or guidance to state legislatures and local school boards considering legislation or policies to ban transgender adolescents from playing sports, inclusive sex education, and teaching racism in the context of US history in schools.

References

1. Sanders RA. Adolescent psychosocial, social, and cognitive development. *Pediatr Rev.* 2013;34(8):354–358 PMID: 23908362 doi: 10.1542/pir.34.8.354
2. Helms JE. Introduction: review of racial identity terminology. In: Helms JE, ed. *Black and White Racial Identity: Theory, Research, and Practice.* Praeger; 1990
3. Rosario M, Schrimshaw EW, Hunter J. Different patterns of sexual identity development over time: implications for the psychological adjustment of lesbian, gay, and bisexual youths. *J Sex Res.* 2011;48(1):3–15 PMID: 19916104 doi: 10.1080/00224490903331067
4. Turban JL, Ehrensaft D. Research review: gender identity in youth: treatment paradigms and controversies. *J Child Psychol Psychiatry.* 2018;59(12):1228–1243 PMID: 29071722 doi: 10.1111/jcpp.12833
5. Crenshaw K. Demarginalizing the intersection of race and sex: a Black feminist critique of antidiscrimination doctrine, feminist theory and antiracist politics. *Univ Chic Leg Forum.* 1989;(1):8

6. Bowleg L. "Once you've blended the cake, you can't take the parts back to the main ingredients": Black gay and bisexual men's descriptions and experiences of intersectionality. *Sex Roles.* 2013;68(11):754–767 doi: 10.1007/s11199-012-0152-4

7. Fields E, Morgan A, Sanders RA. The intersection of sociocultural factors and health-related behavior in lesbian, gay, bisexual, and transgender youth: experiences among young Black gay males as an example. *Pediatr Clin North Am.* 2016;63(6):1091–1106 PMID: 27865335 doi: 10.1016/j.pcl.2016.07.009

8. Rosario M, Schrimshaw EW, Hunter J, Braun L. Sexual identity development among gay, lesbian, and bisexual youths: consistency and change over time. *J Sex Res.* 2006;43(1):46–58 PMID: 16817067 doi: 10.1080/00224490609552298

9. Nesmith AA, Burton DL, Cosgrove TJ. Gay, lesbian, and bisexual youth and young adults: social support in their own words. *J Homosex.* 1999;37(1):95–108 PMID: 10203072 doi: 10.1300/J082v37n01_07

10. Arrington-Sanders R, Hailey-Fair K, Wirtz AL, et al. Role of structural marginalization, HIV stigma, and mistrust on HIV prevention and treatment among young Black Latinx men who have sex with men and transgender women: perspectives from youth service providers. *AIDS Patient Care STDS.* 2020;34(1):7–15 PMID: 31944853 doi: 10.1089/apc.2019.0165

11. Testa RJ, Michaels MS, Bliss W, Rogers ML, Balsam KF, Joiner T. Suicidal ideation in transgender people: gender minority stress and interpersonal theory factors. *J Abnorm Psychol.* 2017;126(1):125–136 PMID: 27831708 doi: 10.1037/abn0000234

12. Meyer IH. Minority stress and mental health in gay men. *J Health Soc Behav.* 1995;36(1):38–56 PMID: 7738327 doi: 10.2307/2137286

13. VanBronkhorst SB, Edwards EM, Roberts DE, et al. Suicidality among psychiatrically hospitalized lesbian, gay, bisexual, transgender, queer, and/or questioning youth: risk and protective factors. *LGBT Health.* 2021;8(6):395–403 PMID: 34424726 doi: 10.1089/lgbt.2020.0278

14. Mills-Koonce WR, Rehder PD, McCurdy AL. The significance of parenting and parent-child relationships for sexual and gender minority adolescents. *J Res Adolesc.* 2018;28(3):637–649 PMID: 30515946 doi: 10.1111/jora.12404

15. Meyer IH, Schwartz S, Frost DM. Social patterning of stress and coping: does disadvantaged social statuses confer more stress and fewer coping resources? *Soc Sci Med.* 2008;67(3):368–379 PMID: 18433961 doi: 10.1016/j.socscimed.2008.03.012

16. Johns MM, Lowry R, Andrzejewski J, et al. Transgender identity and experiences of violence victimization, substance use, suicide risk, and sexual risk behaviors among high school students—19 states and large urban school districts, 2017. *MMWR Morb Mortal Wkly Rep.* 2019;68(3):67–71 PMID: 30677012 doi: 10.15585/mmwr.mm6803a3

17. Ransome Y, Kawachi I, Braunstein S, Nash D. Structural inequalities drive late HIV diagnosis: the role of black racial concentration, income inequality, socioeconomic deprivation, and HIV testing. *Health Place.* 2016;42:148–158 PMID: 27770671 doi: 10.1016/j.healthplace.2016.09.004

18. Arrington-Sanders R, Alvarenga A, Galai N, et al. Social determinants of transactional sex in a sample of young Black and Latinx sexual minority cisgender men and transgender women. *J Adolesc Health.* 2022;70(2):275–281 PMID: 34580030 doi: 10.1016/j.jadohealth.2021.08.002

19. Velez BL, Cox R, Polihronakis CJ, Moradi B. Discrimination, work outcomes, and mental health among women of color: the protective role of womanist attitudes. *J Couns Psychol.* 2018;65(2):178–193 PMID: 29543474 doi: 10.1037/cou0000274

CHAPTER 10

The Intersection of Racism, Immigration, and Child Health

Diana Montoya-Williams, MD, MSHP; Julie M. Linton, MD;
and Olanrewaju Falusi, MD, MEd

Introduction

Immigration is a critical aspect of life and society in the United States. Factors such as one's nativity (ie, where one is born), the migration journey, and one's immigration status are crucial social determinants of health that affect legal, logistic, cultural, and language access to health insurance and health care. This differential access creates health inequities rooted in local, state, and federal immigration policies and practices.[1] This chapter defines terms needed to understand relationships between immigration, racism, and child health; provides an overview of how immigration policies contribute to racially founded child health inequities; and offers recommendations to mitigate structural racism and discrimination against immigrant children and families.

Current and Historical Foundational Concepts

In 2019, nearly 45 million immigrants were living in the United States, or 13.7% of the population. Children who were born outside the country or who have at least one parent who was born outside the country currently represent 1 in 4 US children.[2] Attitudes toward immigrants and, by extension, immigration policies contribute to structural discrimination through racism, colorism, xenophobia, nativism, or religious discrimination (Box 10–1). Discriminatory attitudes, policies, and practices affect access to quality care and, ultimately, the health and well-being of immigrant children.

The history of US immigration policy embodies structural racism, colorism, and xenophobia (Table 10–1). The first US immigration law, the Naturalization Act of 1790, provided that "free white persons" living in the United States for at least 2 years were eligible for citizenship,[3] racializing US immigration policy from the outset. Designation of "un-desirable" immigrants based on national origin began in 1875, targeting Chinese laborers, people involved in the criminal justice system, and commercial sex workers.[4] Inequitable policies persisted throughout the 20th century. The 1921 Emergency Quota Act deliberately favored immigrants from northwestern Europe,[4] and in the 1960s, Cuban refugees, many of whom were wealthy, well educated, and light skinned, received preferential access to lawful status.[3,5] In contrast, after 1965, with the termination of the temporary Bracero Agreement labor program and new policies capping the number of permanent resident visas, paths to legal immigration and residence were curtailed or eliminated for those who had or wished to emigrate from Central America. As a result, the number of undocumented Mexican immigrants rose.[6] Starting in 2017, federal policies, including the Muslim ban (Executive Order 13769), the zero-tolerance policy (Executive Order 13841), termination of the Deferred Action for Childhood Arrivals program, and the public charge regulation, disproportionately harmed families from Central America, Africa, and the Middle East, most of whom are people of color.[7]

Box 10–1.

Foundational Concepts

Racism

Systematic structuring of opportunity and application of value in favor of some races over others, with an understanding that race is a socially constructed representation of groups of people who share physical or social attributes

Colorism

Discriminatory practices that show preference for lighter skin tones, straight hair, and more Eurocentric facial features

Xenophobia

Prejudice against or fear of people from other countries

Nativism

Policies that demonstrate protection of or favor for native inhabitants rather than immigrants

Religious Discrimination

Discriminatory practices against an individual's or group's religious beliefs and practices and/or their request for accommodations of their religious beliefs and practices

Further, immigration policy research has inadequately examined the effect of structural racism on immigrants' health because race and ethnicity are not recorded by federal immigration administrations and are often conflated.[8] This inadequacy is exemplified by the policies and practices leading to family separation. Historically, the discriminatory quotas in 1921 provided no exemptions for people trying to reunite with family members already residing within the United States. In addition, the 1924 National Origins Quota Act (Table 10–1) exempted only immediate family members of US citizens, preventing many extended or multigenerational refugee families, such as Armenian and Jewish people, from reuniting.[9] Recently, during the execution of the zero-tolerance policy in 2018, the sentinel family-separation case (the *Ms. L v ICE* case) involved a mother and daughter from the Democratic Republic of the Congo.[10] However, national discourse underemphasized the role of structural racism in the design and execution of this policy.

Policies of exclusion have also incorporated public health conditions and experiences that have disproportionately affected communities of color, contributing to structural racism. In 1891, the federal government began requiring medical officers from the Public Health Service to exclude immigrants with infectious diseases and chronic conditions, including serious mental illnesses, intellectual disabilities, and epilepsy.[11] On Ellis Island, mass examinations disproportionately excluded immigrants from Asia and Central America.[11] Recently, in 2019, the federal administration broadened the definition of a public charge to include people who have used anti-poverty programs such as Medicaid, the Supplemental Nutrition Assistance Program, and public housing.[12] This rule was reversed in 2021; however, its chilling effect had already triggered decreased enrollment in federal benefit programs.[13] By restricting participation in public programs designed to keep people healthy, expansion of the public charge rule codified limitations on one's ability to reach optimal health and financial security. It also targeted immigrants more likely to experience poverty, disproportionately and structurally discriminating against communities of color.

Immigration Enforcement and Racism

Despite the discriminatory redefinition of who qualifies for admission into the United States, the rates and diversity of immigration have risen significantly since the

Table 10–1. A Select Timeline of Key Policies Highlighting the Intersection of Racism and Immigration		
Year	Act	Description
1790	Naturalization Act of 1790	"Free white persons" living in the United States for at least 2 years were eligible for citizenship
1798	Alien and Sedition Acts	Authorized the president to deport immigrants without citizenship when deemed "dangerous to the peace and safety of the United States"
1882	Chinese Exclusion Act	Banned immigration of Chinese laborers, prevented naturalization of and permitted removal of Chinese immigrants
	Immigration Act of 1882	

(continued on next page)

Table 10–1 (*continued*)		
Year	**Act**	**Description**
1921	Emergency Quota Act	Placed first numerical cap on admissions that was based on nationality
1924	National Origins Quota Act	Made national origin the basis for admission into the United States
1942	Bracero Agreement	Allowed Mexican nationals to migrate to the United States as temporary agricultural workers
1948	Displaced Persons Act	Created a national displaced persons policy
1962	Migration and Refugee Assistance Act of 1962	Allocated funds to people fleeing to the western hemisphere from countries of origin because of persecution or fear of persecution based on race, religion, or political opinion
1965	Immigration and Nationality Act of 1965	Eliminated the national origin system and replaced it with an emphasis on family-based immigration
1980	Refugee Act of 1980	Established a new system to process and admit refugees fleeing from overseas and those seeking asylum in the United States or at US borders

Table 10–1 (*continued*)		
Year	**Act**	**Description**
1996	Personal Responsibility and Work Opportunity Reconciliation Act of 1996	Excluded many immigrants from participation in public programs
2012	Deferred Action for Childhood Arrivals	Deferred action policy that shields some undocumented immigrants who came to the United States as children from deportation and provides them with work authorization
2017	Muslim ban	A presidential executive order banning travel from 7 predominantly Muslim countries (Iran, Iraq, Libya, Somalia, Sudan, Syria, and Yemen) and suspending Syrian refugee resettlement
2018	Zero-tolerance/family separation policy	Criminally prosecuted all migrants entering the United States without authorization, leading to the separation of children from their families
2019	Public charge rule change	Broadened the existing definition of a public charge to include people who have used anti-poverty programs such as Medicaid, the Supplemental Nutrition Assistance Program, and public housing. This new rule was reversed in 2021.

Immigration and Nationality Act of 1965, which abolished quotas based on national origin. Simultaneously, immigration enforcement by immigration officials has evolved to prioritize detention and deportation. Since the 1990s, expanded militarization at the border, expedited deportations, and residential and work site raids have increased the criminalization of immigrants, particularly those who are undocumented.[14,15] Federal 287(g) programs, in 24 states as of January 2023, extend the reach of Immigration and

Customs Enforcement by allowing local and state authorities to act as immigration enforcement agents who can detain undocumented immigrants.

Across federal, state, and local jurisdictions, disproportionate policing of Black people results in larger numbers of Black immigrants being detained and deported. Between 2003 and 2015, Black immigrants made up 5.4% of the overall undocumented population in the United States but represented 10.6% of all immigrants in removal proceedings. In 2015, Black immigrants made up 7.2% of all immigrants without citizenship yet made up 20.3% of immigrants in deportation proceedings.[16] There is no evidence that Black immigrants commit crimes at greater rates than other immigrants; these disparities indicate systemic anti-Blackness within the immigration legal system. This bias was displayed in September 2021 as US border agents forcibly removed Haitian migrants at the US-Mexico border, sometimes yielding whiplike cords.[17] Additional immigrant groups that are adversely affected by racial profiling and enforcement include Latin American, South Asian, Middle Eastern, and Muslim communities, an effect further deepening inequities between immigrants of color and white immigrants, and, more broadly, white Americans.[8,18]

Immigration Policy and Child Health Inequities

Immigrant disparities in child health outcomes illustrate the adverse legacy of ongoing policy inequities. Children in immigrant families are more likely to be uninsured, including 10% of citizen children with a noncitizen parent, 17% of lawfully present immigrant children (including refugees), and 28% of undocumented children (including unaccompanied immigrant children), than the 4% of citizen children with citizen parents.[19] This inequity leaves children who may experience greater medical and mental health needs without consistent access to care.[20] Additionally, children in immigrant families experience disparate poverty rates compared with children in nonimmigrant families (20.9% vs 9.9%).[20] However, they benefit less or are excluded from critical anti-poverty programs, including the Earned Income Tax Credit program, the Child Tax Credit program, and the Supplemental Nutrition Assistance Program.[2] Finally, increased immigration enforcement has been linked to adverse child health outcomes. For instance, the 2017 Muslim ban was associated with preterm births among women from banned countries[21] and immigration raids have been associated with increased rates of low birth weights among Hispanic women.[22]

The Role of Data in Dismantling Immigration-Related Racism

Through research, public health, and quality improvement, pediatric health professionals can collect disaggregated data that better reflect risk profiles. This data can elucidate, for instance, how the health of individuals born outside the United States and emigrating from different regions or Indigenous cultures of Latin America differs in response to changing immigration policies, as well as how structural racism and colorism affect the health of immigrant Asian or Black subgroups. Widespread collection of disaggregated data will facilitate multisite research and quality improvement that can help overcome statistical challenges when studying disaggregated groups.[23] Pediatric health professionals can consider collecting nativity data in addition to race and ethnicity data to create demographic categories that capture intersecting racially minoritized dimensions (eg, "Hispanic Black person born outside the United States"). Other frameworks for patient descriptors may also be useful. For instance, the framework PROGRESS-Plus (**P**lace of residence, **R**ace/ethnicity/culture/language, **O**ccupation, **G**ender/sex, **R**eligion, **E**ducation, **S**ocioeconomic status, and **S**ocial capital, **Plus** other personal and relational features such as sexual orientation, disability, age, immigration status, and educational attainment) offers a more comprehensive approach.[24]

To fully understand the intersection of racism, immigration, and child health, it is essential to examine how data on race, ethnicity, and language preference has been collected, given well-documented inaccuracies, particularly within electronic health records.[24] Equally important is using data to document structural racism and xenophobia. For example, indices that score states' structural xenophobia[1] or data sets that analyze immigrant sanctuary policies[25] are examples of tools to go beyond the examination of race, ethnicity, and nativity on an individual level to the examination of societal structures instead.

Summary

The complex and racist history of US immigration policy and enforcement threatens the health and well-being of children in immigrant families. Through clinical, educational, research, and advocacy strategies, pediatric health professionals can help advance health equity for all children in immigrant families.

Recommendations

Patient- and Family-Directed

- Use trained interpreters in all encounters for families who prefer languages other than English.
- Screen for social determinants of health, including immigration-related issues.
- Provide trauma-informed care that acknowledges immigration-related trauma.

- Address the unique health needs of unaccompanied immigrant children who have been reunited with sponsors in communities.

- Consider language access when making referrals, including the process by which patients schedule appointments.

- Engage in ongoing personal education to deliver care that embodies cultural humility and safety.

Clinical Practice/Organizations/Systems

- Systematically train all team members to effectively engage with interpreters and confirm bilingual and multilingual staff's fluency through formalized language testing.

- Create inclusive health care environments that explicitly welcome immigrants, such as welcoming signage (eg, "All are welcome") in languages that represent patient populations.

- Educate and prepare staff about immigrants' rights concerning immigration enforcement.

- Query accuracy of race, ethnicity, and language data collection within electronic health records.

- Collect disaggregated data, informed by frameworks such as PROGRESS-Plus, that better identify characteristics driving health inequities.[26]

- Support cross-sectoral collaborations with sociologists, political scientists, and demographic researchers to better measure the effect of structural racism and xenophobia on immigrant health.

- Develop medicolegal partnerships in the clinical space or as external referrals to connect families with a path to stable legal status.

- Create paid family advisory boards that include families with preferences for languages other than English.

Public Health Policy and Community Advocacy

- Engage with professional organizations with advocacy agendas to enhance collective impact.

- Contribute to state-based efforts to expand insurance coverage for immigrant children.

- Participate in local, state, and national coalitions to protect immigrant families' civil rights.

- Authentically engage with local neighborhoods by participating in or creating community-based events sponsored by your institution.

- Work with and amplify the work of local community-based immigrant advocacy groups.

References

1. Samari G, Nagle A, Coleman-Minahan K. Measuring structural xenophobia: US state immigration policy climates over ten years. *SSM Popul Health.* 2021;16:100938 PMID: 34660879 doi: 10.1016/j. ssmph.2021.100938
2. Linton JM, Green A, Chilton LA, et al; American Academy of Pediatrics Council on Community Pediatrics. Providing care for children in immigrant families. *Pediatrics.* 2019;144(3):e20192077 PMID: 31427460 doi: 10.1542/peds.2019-2077
3. Migration Policy Institute. *Major US Immigration Laws, 1790-Present.* Migration Policy Institute; 2013. https://www.migrationpolicy.org/sites/default/files/publications/CIR-1790Timeline.pdf
4. Ewing WA. Opportunity and exclusion: a brief history of U.S. immigration policy. Immigration Policy Center. January 2012. Accessed February 3, 2023. https://www.americanimmigrationcouncil.org/sites/default/files/research/opportunity_exclusion_011312.pdf
5. Duany J. Cuban migration: a postrevolution exodus ebbs and flows. Migration Policy Institute. July 6, 2017. Accessed February 3, 2023. https://www.migrationpolicy.org/article/cuban-migration-postrevolution-exodus-ebbs-and-flows
6. Massey DS, Pren KA. Unintended consequences of US immigration policy: explaining the post-1965 surge from Latin America. *Popul Dev Rev.* 2012;38(1):1-29 PMID: 22833862 doi: 10.1111/j.1728-4457.2012.00470.x
7. Srikantiah J, Sinnar S. White nationalism as immigration policy. Stanford Law Review. Accessed February 3, 2023. https://www.stanfordlawreview.org/online/white-nationalism-as-immigration-policy
8. Bernstein H, McTarnaghan S, Islam A. Centering race and structural racism in immigration policy research. Urban Institute. December 2021. Accessed February 3, 2023. https://www.urban.org/sites/default/files/publication/105202/centering-race-and-structural-racism-in-immigration-policy-research.pdf
9. Schacher Y. Family separation and lives in limbo: U.S. immigration policy in the 1920s and during the Trump administration. *Ann Am Acad Pol Soc Sci.* 2020;690(1):192-199 doi: 10.1177/0002716220941571
10. Ms. L v. ICE. American Civil Liberties Union. Accessed February 3, 2023. https://www.aclu.org/legal-document/ms-l-v-ice-complaint
11. Fairchild AL. Policies of inclusion: immigrants, disease, dependency, and American immigration policy at the dawn and dusk of the 20th century. *Am J Public Health.* 2004;94(4):528-539 PMID: 15053996 doi: 10.2105/AJPH.94.4.528
12. Barofsky J, Vargas A, Rodriguez D, Barrows A. Spreading fear: the announcement of the public charge rule reduced enrollment in child safety-net programs. *Health Aff (Millwood).* 2020;39(10):1752-1761 PMID: 33017237 doi: 10.1377/hlthaff.2020.00763
13. Haley JM, Kenney GM, Bernstein H, Gonzalez D. Many immigrant families with children continued to avoid public benefits in 2020, despite facing hardships. Urban Institute. May 26, 2021. Accessed February 3, 2023. https://www.urban.org/research/publication/many-immigrant-families-children-continued-avoid-public-benefits-2020-despite-facing-hardships
14. Aranda E, Vaquera E. Racism, the immigration enforcement regime, and the implications for racial inequality in the lives of undocumented young adults. *Sociol Race Ethn (Thousand Oaks).* 2015;1(1):88-104 doi: 10.1177/2332649214551097
15. Ramón C, Cardinal Brown T. Decriminalizing illegal border crossing: what does it mean? an explainer of civil vs. criminal immigration enforcement. Bipartisan Policy Center. January 15, 2020. Accessed February 3, 2023. https://bipartisanpolicy.org/blog/decriminalizing-illegal-border-crossing-what-does-it-mean-an-explainer-of-civil-vs-criminal-immigration-enforcement
16. Morgan-Trostle J, Zheng K, Lipscombe C. *The State of Black Immigrants.* Black Alliance for Just Immigration, NYU School of Law Immigrant Rights Clinic; 2022

17. Sullivan E, Kanno-Youngs Z. Images of border patrol's treatment of Haitian migrants prompt outrage. *New York Times.* September 22, 2021. Accessed February 3, 2023. https://www.nytimes.com/2021/09/21/us/politics/haitians-border-patrol-photos.html

18. Modi R. *Communities on Fire: Confronting Hate Violence and Xenophobic Political Rhetoric.* South Asian Americans Leading Together; 2018. Accessed February 3, 2023. https://saalt.org/wp-content/uploads/2018/01/Communities-on-Fire.pdf

19. Health coverage and care of immigrants. Kaiser Family Foundation. December 20, 2022. Accessed February 3, 2023. https://www.kff.org/racial-equity-and-health-policy/fact-sheet/health-coverage-of-immigrants

20. Acevedo-Garcia D, Joshi PK, Ruskin E, Walters AN, Sofer N, Guevara CA. Including children in immigrant families in policy approaches to reduce child poverty. *Acad Pediatr.* 2021;21(8)(suppl):S117–S125 PMID: 34740418 doi: 10.1016/j.acap.2021.06.016

21. Samari G, Catalano R, Alcalá HE, Gemmill A. The Muslim ban and preterm birth: analysis of U.S. vital statistics data from 2009 to 2018. *Soc Sci Med.* 2020;265:113544 PMID: 33261902 doi: 10.1016/j.socscimed.2020.113544

22. Novak NL, Geronimus AT, Martinez-Cardoso AM. Change in birth outcomes among infants born to Latina mothers after a major immigration raid. *Int J Epidemiol.* 2017;46(3):839–849 PMID: 28115577

23. Montoya-Williams D, Peña MM, Fuentes-Afflick E. In pursuit of health equity in pediatrics. *J Pediatr X.* 2020;5:100045 PMID: 33733084 doi: 10.1016/j.ympdx.2020.100045

24. Reichman V, Brachio SS, Madu CR, Montoya-Williams D, Peña MM. Using rising tides to lift all boats: equity-focused quality improvement as a tool to reduce neonatal health disparities. *Semin Fetal Neonatal Med.* 2021;26(1):101198 PMID: 33558160 doi: 10.1016/j.siny.2021.101198

25. Ortiz R, Farrell-Bryan D, Gutierrez G, et al. A content analysis of US sanctuary immigration policies: implications for research in social determinants of health. *Health Aff (Millwood).* 2021;40(7):1145–1153 PMID: 34228526 doi: 10.1377/hlthaff.2021.00097

26. Officer CE. PROGRESS-Plus. Cochrane Methods Equity. Accessed February 3, 2023. https://methods.cochrane.org/equity/projects/evidence-equity/progress-plus

CHAPTER 11

Neurodevelopmental Disorders and the Impact of Racism

Adiaha Spinks-Franklin, MD, MPH; Shruti Mittal, MD; Silvia Pereira-Smith, MD; and Nathaniel Beers, MD, MPA

Introduction

The impact of racism has led to significant disparities in the diagnosis and management of neurodevelopmental disorders (NDDs) in Black, Indigenous, and People of Color (BIPOC) youth (children, adolescents, and young adults). Many NDD diagnoses, such as attention-deficit/hyperactivity disorder (ADHD), learning disorders (LDs), and autism spectrum disorder (ASD), are overdiagnosed, misdiagnosed, or under-identified in BIPOC youth compared with other medical conditions (eg, asthma, diabetes). These disparities influence the types and quality of services received, leading to long-term negative effects.

Overdiagnosis

Several factors contribute to the overdiagnosis of NDDs in BIPOC youth, such as implicit racial biases of educators and pediatric health professionals, exposure to adverse childhood experiences (ACEs), and the impact of toxic stress on families who have experienced racism.

Implicit racial biases of educators and pediatric health professionals can play a significant role in the overdiagnosis of NDDs in BIPOC youth. For example, the diagnosis of ADHD depends on teacher feedback, therapist feedback, pediatric health professional observations, and parent/caregiver or family reports. All of these sources are subject to significant bias related to race. Studies using eye-tracking technology have shown that in preschool settings, when children engage in typical activities, educators look at Black boys longer than white children, suggesting an expectation of more challenging behavior.[1] Although evidence suggests that there may be no difference in the true incidence of ADHD among cultural and racial groups, younger Black children are more likely to be diagnosed with ADHD than younger Latine[a] and younger white children.[2]

Teachers often misinterpret the behaviors of BIPOC students to be hostile or threatening and therefore penalize them with harsher punishments. Although Black students make up only 19% of preschool enrollment, they make up 47% of preschoolers who receive suspensions.[1] Additionally, Black girls receive suspensions from school at 6 times

---

[a]In this chapter, we use *Latine* when referring to people of Latin American origin or descent as a whole. It is a gender-neutral and gender-inclusive alternative to *Latino*. For a brief history of this term, including a rationale, refer to the book introduction.

the rate of their white counterparts for the same behaviors.[3] In fact, students with multiple marginalized intersecting identities have the highest rate of harsh school punishment and are more frequently funneled into the School-Prison Nexus (also referred to as the "school-to-prison pipeline"). The School-Prison Nexus refers to the active targeting of marginalized students for harsh school punishment practices that place them at high risk for contact with the criminal legal system.[4] The special education system plays a central role by which students with multiple marginalized identities come in early contact with the juvenile legal system. School officials are twice as likely to harshly punish economically poor, BIPOC students with NDDs who receive special education services than their peers with similar offenses. These harsh punishments include out-of-school suspensions, expulsions, corporal punishment (allowed for students with disabilities in 19 states), and referrals to law enforcement agencies, all of which increase their risk for contact with the juvenile legal system.[5] Specifically, Black and American Indian/Alaska Native boys with disabilities receiving special education service have the highest rates of suspension, expulsion, corporal punishment, and referral to law enforcement.[6] This disproportionality of harsh punishment of BIPOC students with NDDs within the special education system contributes to poor educational outcomes, increased risk of dropping out of high school, and ongoing contact with the criminal legal system.

The effects of racism and ACEs on family members also contribute to the overdiagnosis of ADHD and other externalizing disorders in BIPOC children, who are misdiagnosed with conduct disorder and disruptive behavior disorders more frequently than white children with similar behavior profiles.[7] Exposure to 4 or more ACEs is associated with an increased risk for learning and behavior differences.[8] Children who experience toxic stress in early childhood can often present with poorly controlled impulses and challenged executive functioning that, together, resemble ADHD symptoms; however, determining the root cause of a child's behaviors is crucial. Black parents who endure more racial discrimination rate ADHD behaviors as higher in their sons.[9] After adjustment for demographic and socioeconomic factors, exposure to racism increased the odds of a child being diagnosed with ADHD by 3.2%.[10] Within special education systems, BIPOC youth are often misclassified as being eligible for special education services under the classification of *intellectual disability* or *emotional disability* rather than as having another NDD, such as ADHD, a speech/language disorder, or a specific LD, such as dyslexia.[11]

Under-identification and Delayed Diagnosis

A common occurrence regarding NDDs in BIPOC youth is under-identification and delayed diagnosis. Black students (and, to a lesser extent, Latine students) are less likely to be diagnosed with an LD than white students,[12] whereas Native American students are often misdiagnosed with an intellectual disability instead of correctly diagnosed with an LD. Neurodevelopmental disorders may be missed in Asian American students because of implicit racial biases of pediatric health professionals based on the model minority myth (refer to Chapter 8, The Model Minority Myth and Chapter 11,

Neurodevelopmental Disorders and the Impact of Racism), a stereotype that generalizes Asian Americans as intelligent and conscientious. Misinformation can also negatively affect diagnostic clarity (eg, a speech delay can be better explained by bilingualism or by not diagnosing a language disorder in the presence of bilingualism or misdiagnosing a speech delay in the presence of a language such as Ebonics [a form of Africanized American English] or Gullah). Regarding ASD, Black children tend to be diagnosed with ADHD and other externalizing disorders first, which leads to a delayed diagnosis of ASD, whereas Latine and Asian American children are initially given diagnoses in speech and global developmental delays.[13] Parents/caregivers of autistic Black children have noted trepidations about primary health professionals who ignore early concerns regarding their child's developmental delays; many report that racial bias has negatively influenced the caregiver–primary health professional interactions.[14] Black and Latine parents are less likely than white parents to report that their health professional spent enough time with their child and showed sensitivity to their family's values.[15]

Diagnostic delays occur for undocumented immigrant children in the United States because they are ineligible for federal health care programs. Without adequate insurance coverage, immigrant families may choose to forego health supervision visits and subspecialty care. Medical homes are critical for trained health professionals to perform regular surveillance and screening for NDDs, yet BIPOC children experience decreased access to them because of systemic barriers.[16] Although most pediatric health professionals provide routine developmental screening as recommended by the American Academy of Pediatrics, significantly fewer offer it in a language other than English, even though free screening measures exist in multiple languages.[17] Health care systems do not consistently support navigation of services in languages other than English, a structural barrier for families with emerging English proficiency.

There are ethnocultural differences in expectations of achievement related to developmental milestones, including personal and social milestones,[18] which influence perceptions of behaviors related to NDDs and may influence when and how a caregiver endorses concerns. Caregivers may be less likely to pathologize a child's behavioral issues because of cultural differences in what constitutes a disability (eg, Arab immigrant Muslim mothers were noted to report disruptive behaviors in their child but not attribute them as symptoms of ADHD).[19]

Disparities in Provision of Services

Black students and multilingual students are overrepresented in special education systems for behavior challenges and other subjective reasons, yet they are significantly less likely to receive services and interventions to address their NDDs.[10,20] Meanwhile, Asian American students are underrepresented in special education and overrepresented in gifted and talented programs.[20] Youth who are misclassified in special education systems receive less appropriate therapeutic interventions, such as reading support for a specific LD.

Pediatricians with negative implicit racial biases are less likely to ask Black caregivers and multilingual caregivers about their concerns regarding their child's development even when their child is likely to experience an NDD.[21] Pediatricians are less likely to refer BIPOC youth at risk for NDDs for early intervention (EI).[22] Those referred for EI are less likely to undergo a developmental evaluation.[22] Latine patients who reported experiencing racial discrimination in a health care setting were less likely to seek preventive care or follow the physician's recommendations.[23] BIPOC youth are significantly less likely to receive medical or behavioral treatment for their ADHD,[22] a finding that suggests reduced access to appropriate health care, physician racial bias, and caregiver perceptions/mistrust of the medical system.

Summary

To change the paradigm, pediatric health professionals and educators must approach all youth as individuals, not as representatives of specific racial or ethnic stereotypes. There are many actions that pediatric health professionals can take to decrease the role of racism in the diagnosis and management of NDDs, including recognizing and mitigating the ways in which our own implicit racial biases influence our practices and being respectful of cultural perspectives in the perception of illness, plus implications of racism, toxic stress, and ACEs on parenting/caregiving and child development.

Recommendations

Patient- and Family-Directed

- Empower families by encouraging them to share their concerns, then respond accordingly.

- Understand that experiences with maltreatment in health care settings could contribute to the underreporting of concerns (eg, for fear of being reported to the child protection system) and to the various cultural perspectives that may result in the overreporting or underreporting of concerns. Listen to caregiver concerns and use objective, systematic methods of eliciting concerns.

- Subjectivity and ambiguity lead to bias-based behaviors in health professionals. Be aware of your own negative racial biases when creating treatment plans and referrals. Create practice systems and protocols that can reduce the likelihood of engaging in bias-based behaviors (eg, automatically refer youth with failed developmental screening results for EI regardless of sociodemographic category).

- Use standardized, language-appropriate screening tools consistently for all patients to prevent biased observations and reporting.

- Provide developmentally appropriate and culturally informed anticipatory guidance, which includes leveraging resources within schools such as individual learning plans with accommodations that are tailored to the student's needs.

- Consider the language needs of the family in providing care and making referrals for services.
- Encourage shared decision-making to empower the patient and family to drive management goals.
- Ask caregivers about the role that racism and other forms of discrimination play in their lives and about how their caregiving has been affected by discrimination.

Clinical Practice/Organizations/Systems

- Ensure that peer support and parent/caregiver navigator models are available to assist patients and families in accessing services in health care, education, and other community agencies.
- Train child care providers and school staff on the role that racial bias plays in identifying and treating NDDs.
- Advocate for developmentally appropriate and culturally informed behavioral management in schools that focuses on removing racial and ethnic biases and eliminating zero-tolerance policies that disproportionately punish Black, Latine, and Native American students.
- Advocate for early, systematic developmental screening for NDDs with data sharing between systems that allows for a reduction in duplicated efforts. Train medical students, residents, and community pediatric health professionals on the role that racial bias and racism play in identifying and treating NDDs, using nationally recognized tools for medical professionals, such as
  - The Association of American Medical Colleges report "Diversity, Equity, and Inclusion Competencies Across the Learning Continuum" (www.aamc.org/data-reports/report/diversity-equity-and-inclusion-competencies-across-learning-continuum)
  - The American Board of Pediatrics Entrustable Professional Activity 14 for General Pediatrics "Use Population Health Strategies and Quality Improvement Methods to Promote Health and Address Racism, Discrimination, and Other Contributors to Inequities Among Pediatric Populations" (www.abp.org/news/press-releases/entrustable-professional-activity-revised-set-anti-racism-professional-standard)
  - The American Council on Graduate Medical Education initiative *ACGME Equity Matters* (www.acgme.org/initiatives/diversity-equity-and-inclusion/ACGME-Equity-Matters)

Public Health Policy and Community Advocacy

- Advocate for school funding models that change public school funding inequities, considering historical underfunding and disenfranchisement of schools in BIPOC communities.

- Advocate for accurate reporting of disorders and disciplinary and punishment actions in schools by race and ethnicity.
- Increase the number of racially, ethnically, linguistically diverse teachers and school staff to align with student demographics.
- Advocate for college loan repayment programs that could help reduce the economic challenges that many BIPOC college students face and that would not dissuade them from going into careers in education.

References

1. Gilliam WS, Maupin AN, Reyes CR, Accavitti M, Shic F. *Do Early Educators' Implicit Biases Regarding Sex and Race Relate to Behavior Expectations and Recommendations of Preschool Expulsions and Suspensions?* Yale University Child Study Center; 2016

2. Zablotsky B, Alford JM. Racial and ethnic differences in the prevalence of attention-deficit/hyperactivity disorder and learning disabilities among U.S. children aged 3–17 years. *NCHS Data Brief.* 2020;(358):1–8 PMID: 32487288

3. Williams Crenshaw K. *Black Girls Matter: Pushed Out, Overpoliced, and Underprotected.* African American Policy Reform, Center for Intersectionality and Social Policy Studies; 2015

4. Skiba RJ, Arredondo MI, Williams NT. More than a metaphor: the contribution of exclusionary discipline to a school-to-prison pipeline. *Equity Excell Educ.* 2014;47(4):546–564 doi: 10.1080/10665684.2014.958965

5. Annamma S, Morrison D, Jackson D. Disproportionality fills in the gaps: connections between achievement, discipline and special education in the school-to-prison pipeline. *Berkeley Rev Educ.* 2014;5(1) doi: 10.5070/B85110003

6. Office for Civil Rights. *An Overview of Exclusionary Discipline Practices in Public Schools for the 2017-18 School Year.* US Dept of Education; 2021. Accessed May 25, 2023. https://www2.ed.gov/about/offices/list/ocr/docs/crdc-exclusionary-school-discipline.pdf

7. Fadus MC, Ginsburg KR, Sobowale K, et al. Unconscious bias and the diagnosis of disruptive behavior disorders and ADHD in African American and Hispanic youth. *Acad Psychiatry.* 2020;44(1):95–102 PMID: 31713075 doi: 10.1007/s40596-019-01127-6

8. Burke Harris N. The devastating, underdiagnosed toll of toxic stress on children. PBS NewsHour. February 23, 2018. Accessed February 6, 2023. https://www.pbs.org/newshour/show/the-devastating-underdiagnosed-toll-of-toxic-stress-on-children

9. Kang S, Harvey EA. Racial differences between Black parents' and white teachers' perceptions of attention-deficit/hyperactivity disorder behavior. *J Abnorm Child Psychol.* 2020;48(5):661–672 PMID: 31792658 doi: 10.1007/s10802-019-00600-y

10. Anderson AT, Luartz L, Heard-Garris N, Widaman K, Chung PJ. The detrimental influence of racial discrimination on child health in the United States. *J Natl Med Assoc.* 2020;112(4):411–422 PMID: 32532525 doi: 10.1016/j.jnma.2020.04.012

11. Maydosz A. Disproportional representation of minorities in special education. *J Multicult Educ.* 2014;8(2):81–88 doi: 10.1108/JME-01-2014-0002

12. Morgan PL, Farkas G, Hillemeier MM, et al. Minorities are disproportionately underrepresented in special education: longitudinal evidence across five disability conditions. *Educ Res.* 2015;44(5):278–292 PMID: 27445414 doi: 10.3102/0013189X15591157

13. Stahmer AC, Vejnoska S, Iadarola S, et al. Caregiver voices: cross-cultural input on improving access to autism services. *J Racial Ethn Health Disparities.* 2019;6(4):752–773 PMID: 30859514 doi: 10.1007/s40615-019-00575-y

14. Dababnah S, Shaia WE, Campion K, Nichols HM. "We had to keep pushing": caregivers' perspectives on autism screening and referral practices of Black children in primary care. *Intellect Dev Disabil.* 2018;56(5):321–336 PMID: 30273522 doi: 10.1352/1934-9556-56.5.321

15. Magaña S, Parish SL, Son E. Have racial and ethnic disparities in the quality of health care relationships changed for children with developmental disabilities and ASD? *Am J Intellect Dev Disabil.* 2015;120(6):504–513 PMID: 26505871 doi: 10.1352/1944-7558-120.6.504

16. Weller BE, Faubert SJ, Ault AK. Youth access to medical homes and medical home components by race and ethnicity. *Matern Child Health J.* 2020;24(2):241–249 PMID: 31828575 doi: 10.1007/s10995-019-02831-3

17. Zuckerman KE, Mattox KM, Sinche BK, Blaschke GS, Bethell C. Racial, ethnic, and language disparities in early childhood developmental/behavioral evaluations: a narrative review. *Clin Pediatr (Phila).* 2014;53(7):619–631 PMID: 24027231 doi: 10.1177/0009922813501378

18. Pachter LM, Dworkin PH. Maternal expectations about normal child development in 4 cultural groups. *Arch Pediatr Adolesc Med.* 1997;151(11):1144–1150 PMID: 9369877 doi: 10.1001/archpedi.1997.02170480074011

19. AlAzzam M, Daack-Hirsch S. Arab immigrant Muslim mothers' perceptions of children's attention deficit hyperactivity disorder. *Procedia Soc Behav Sci.* 2015;185:23–34 doi: 10.1016/j.sbspro.2015.03.454

20. Ortogero SP, Ray AB. Overrepresentation of English learners in special education amid the COVID-19 pandemic. *Educ Media Int.* 2021;58(2):161–180 doi: 10.1080/09523987.2021.1930485

21. Schnierle J, Christian-Brathwaite N, Louisias M. Implicit bias: what every pediatrician should know about the effect of bias on health and future directions. *Curr Probl Pediatr Adolesc Health Care.* 2019;49(2):34–44 PMID: 30738896 doi: 10.1016/j.cppeds.2019.01.003

22. Breland HL, Ellis C. Perceived discrimination in healthcare settings among Latinos with limited English proficiency in South Carolina. *South Med J.* 2015;108(4):203–206 PMID: 25871985 doi: 10.14423/SMJ.0000000000000259

23. Coker TR, Elliott MN, Toomey SL, et al. Racial and ethnic disparities in ADHD diagnosis and treatment. *Pediatrics.* 2016;138(3):e20160407 PMID: 27553219 doi: 10.1542/peds.2016-0407

Addressing the Impact of Racism on the Mental Health of Youth: A Focus on Pediatric Health Professionals and Collaborators

Alfiee M. Breland-Noble, PhD, MHSc; Bridget E. Weller, PhD; Akilah Patterson, MPH; and Riana Elyse Anderson, PhD, LCP

Introduction

Racism in all forms, including racial discrimination, historical racism, structural oppression, and institutional discrimination, has well-documented negative effects on the mental health of children and adolescents. Children's, adolescents', and young adults' experiences with racism can be acute or chronic, as well as direct or vicarious. Regardless of how racism is experienced, it is associated with mental health outcomes, including suicidal ideation, depression, anxiety, substance misuse, and behavioral issues. In this chapter, we detail the effects of racism on the mental health of youth of color from birth to 25 years of age and provide recommendations for pediatric health professionals and collaborators to mitigate the adverse influence of racism on youth mental health (refer to Box 12–1 for the definitions of key terms used in this chapter[1,2]).

Youth Exposure to Racism

Exposure to racism is a pervasive experience for children and adolescents of color.[3,4] Indeed, children as young as 10 years have reported at least one experience with racism in the prior year.[5] Further, 18.4% of youth, aged 13 through 25, reported often or very often having been exposed to racism in their lifetimes.[6] In addition to lifetime exposure, Black or Latinx[a] youth have reported exposure to racism in upwards of 5 incidents per day.[7] These patterns of exposure to racism suggest that youth of color experience racism throughout their development.

Youth of color experience racism from a variety of sources. Youth have direct experiences with racism through interactions with individuals such as caregivers, police, peers, and teachers.[6] For example, among youth who reported incidents of racial discrimination, 80% indicated experiencing them at school.[8] Youth also experience racism through news outlets,[6] via social media,[7,9] in their geographic communities,[7] and while seeking pediatric health care.[10] Youth also have indirect or vicarious exposure to

---

[a] In this chapter, we use *Latinx* when referring to people of Latin American origin or descent as a whole. It is a gender-neutral and gender-inclusive alternative to *Latino*. For a brief history of this term, including a rationale, refer to the book introduction.

racism, such as their caregivers' experience with racism. Indeed, even before birth, studies show a positive correlation between a mother's experience with racism and a child's low birth weight and preterm delivery.[11] Youth are also exposed to racism through a history of oppressive policies and practices.[12] These various sources of racism make a youth susceptible to experiencing racial trauma, which can influence their mental health.

Box 12–1.

Definitions of Key Terms Used in This Chapter

Mental health

According to the American Medical Association,[1] mental health is defined as "a person's emotional, cognitive and psychological well being" and encompasses aspects of illness and wellness. Mental illnesses are health conditions that involve negative changes in emotion, thinking, or behavior and are associated with distress and problems functioning in social, work, or family activities.

Racial trauma

Racial trauma, or *race-based traumatic stress*, refers to the mental and emotional injury caused by encounters with racial bias and ethnic discrimination, racism, and hate crimes. When any individual has experienced an emotionally painful, sudden, and uncontrollable racist encounter, it places them at risk of having a race-based traumatic stress injury.[2]

Influence of Racism on Youth Mental Health

Regardless of the source, research has shown that racism elevates the likelihood that youth of color will experience mental health conditions. In fact, systematic reviews have shown an association between racism and mental health outcomes for youth.[11] And a more recent study of students in grades 9 through 12 showed that perceived racism was associated with self-reported poor mental health.[4] Specifically, research has shown that experiences with racism are associated with both suicidal ideation[13] and the most common mental health issues among youth (ie, depression, anxiety, behavioral issues, and attention-deficit/hyperactivity disorder).[3,6,14] Considering these outcomes, mental health symptoms may be precipitating factors for youth and families seeking health care.

Recommendations for Pediatric Health Professionals

Because of the deleterious effect of racism on youth mental health, pediatric health professionals and collaborators must be equipped to mitigate the adverse influence of racism on youth mental health. This ability is critical because negative experiences in health care settings are well-documented and can exacerbate previous experiences with racism. Further, experiences in health care settings can affect youth help-seeking behaviors and satisfaction with care.[15] Methods that health care settings and pediatric health professionals can use to provide quality care and to positively influence the mental health of youth of color follow.

Culturally Competent and Culturally Humble Professionals

Pediatric health professionals must develop cultural competency to provide quality care that addresses youth experiences with racism. Pediatric health professionals must be inquisitive without being intrusive, that is, curious but not fascinated, and they need to always work to prevent marginalization or belittling of child, adolescent, or family concerns. If a professional finds that their cultural competence is lacking, they can build cultural knowledge by reading, conducting background research, engaging in immersive community events, and participating in professional development training to expand their knowledge and awareness of varied cultural groups.[16]

We encourage pediatric health professionals to approach enhancing their cultural competency through the lens of cultural humility. This approach allows them to seek a deeper understanding of their worldviews and of how their worldviews compare with their patients'. When done well, this practice supports cognitive flexibility, allowing a professional the opportunity to make mistakes and learn from them. As organizations and systems support pediatric health professionals in developing the knowledge, awareness, and skills to collaborate with patients from varied backgrounds, we then increase access to care and work to reduce poor mental health outcomes among youth of color.

Various training efforts have aspired to increase the quantity of pediatric health professionals with cultural competence and pediatric health professionals from historically underserved communities. These efforts train current and future professionals in culturally appropriate, integrated care that emphasizes the best practices in patient-centered approaches.[17] They include professional development in addressing structural and personal barriers to treatment, enhancing trust between patients and professionals, and naming the presence of racism.[18] These efforts intend to expand the network of culturally competent professionals that can address the influence of racism on youth.

Racial Socialization

Health care settings and pediatric health professionals need to support opportunities for racial socialization to provide quality care for youth of color. Research suggests that racial socialization begun in early childhood is an effective active coping mechanism for youth of color and, therefore, a viable interim strategy.[19] Racial socialization, discussed at length in Chapter 4, How Adults Can Promote Positive Racial and Ethnic Identities in the Context of Structural Racism, is a verbal and behavioral communication strategy between caregivers, professionals, and youth that includes positive messages and attitudes about race and racism. Research suggests that caregivers of color feel they must begin racial conversations early in their children's developmental trajectory and continue these conversations through adolescence to prepare their children for the often racially hostile outside world.[19]

As a next step, health care settings and pediatric health professionals must educate themselves on the importance of racial socialization in our society. By optimizing their comfort level with conversations about race and racial socialization, they will be better equipped to create safe clinical spaces for difficult conversations about race. Examples of safe spaces include opportunities wherein youth and families can share their experiences with racism and be validated, physical spaces in which various lived experiences are included, and places in which dialogue about racism can occur among pediatric health professionals. By engaging in culturally humble and competent conversations, pediatric health professionals can empower and encourage caregivers and their colleagues to incorporate racial socialization skills as part of a healthy, holistic approach to caregiving.

Screening and Assessment

Health care settings and pediatric health professionals must also screen for and assess youth experiences with racism. Pediatric health professionals can implement formal assessments through standardized measures, such as the Perceptions of Racism in Children and Youth,[3] which is a standardized assessment of encounters with racism and discrimination. This self-assessment is valid and reliable for youth 14 to 18 years of age.

In addition to assessing for experiences with racism, pediatric health professionals need to screen for and assess mental health conditions across health care settings. For example, they can screen for common mental health issues through The Suicide Behaviors Questionnaire-Revised,[20] the Severity Measure for Depression—Child Age 11–17,[21] and the Severity Measure for Generalized Anxiety Disorder—Child Age 11–17.[22] When using these tools, pediatric health professionals must include the gathered information to inform treatment planning and treatment itself. Otherwise, excluding this content from the treatment, despite gathering it, can cause further harm to youth.

Name the Experience

In addition to implementing formal assessment, pediatric health professionals can create opportunities for youth and families to name their experiences with racism. This approach allows for authentic healing in pediatric mental health and often begins with allowance of the space youth need to name the issues they face without judgment and without the need to "fix" them. Youth and their caregivers must be permitted to share their experiences with racism and discrimination fully and clearly, even if experienced by the professional.

Referral for Behavioral Health Supports

Pediatric health professionals must also be willing and able to provide referrals for behavioral health to ensure that youth receive quality care that addresses racism. If pediatric health professionals feel that the concerns presented fall outside their expertise, a referral to a culturally competent mental health specialist might be in order. There are numerous directories to facilitate this process, including Melanated Therapists, Therapy for Latinx, and Asians for Mental Health, among others.

Recommendations

Clinical Practice/Organizations/Systems

Pediatric health professionals should

- Engage caregivers and youth in racial socialization conversations.
- Encourage youth to express their experiences with racism.
- Actively expand their personal networks of culturally competent professionals.
- Provide culturally relevant, evidence-informed resources to caregivers.
- Approach the care they provide to youth with cultural humility.
- Equip themselves with the knowledge, awareness, and skills to collaborate with patients from varied racial backgrounds.

References

1. American Medical Association. Mental health. Catalog of Topics. Accessed February 9, 2023. https://www.ama-assn.org/topics/mental-health
2. MHA. Racial trauma. Accessed February 9, 2022. https://www.mhanational.org/racial-trauma
3. Pachter LM, Szalacha LA, Bernstein BA, García Coll C. Perceptions of Racism in Children and Youth (PRaCY): properties of a self-report instrument for research on children's health and development. *Ethn Health*. 2010;15(1):33–46 PMID: 20013438 doi: 10.1080/13557850903383196
4. Mpofu JJ, Cooper AC, Ashley C, et al. Perceived racism and demographic, mental health, and behavioral characteristics among high school students during the COVID-19 pandemic—Adolescent Behaviors and Experiences Survey, United States, January–June 2021. *MMWR Suppl.* 2022;71(3):22–27 PMID: 35358163 doi: 10.15585/mmwr.su7103a4
5. McNeil Smith S, Fincham F. Racial discrimination experiences among Black youth: a person-centered approach. *J Black Psychol.* 2016;42(4):300–319 doi: 10.1177/0095798415573315
6. Breland-Noble A; The AAKOMA Project. *The AAKOMA Project's State of Mental Health for Youth of Color: Executive Summary.* The AAKOMA Project; 2022
7. Tynes BM, Willis HA, Stewart AM, Hamilton MW. Race-related traumatic events online and mental health among adolescents of color. *J Adolesc Health.* 2019;65(3):371–377 PMID: 31196779 doi: 10.1016/j.jadohealth.2019.03.006
8. Coker TR, Elliott MN, Kanouse DE, et al. Perceived racial/ethnic discrimination among fifth-grade students and its association with mental health. *Am J Public Health.* 2009;99(5):878–884 PMID: 19299673 doi: 10.2105/AJPH.2008.144329

9. Portillo NL, Grapin SL, Reyes-Portillo JA, Masia Warner C. Online discrimination and mental health outcomes: the moderating roles of ethnic identity and immigrant generation among Latinx young adults. *J Lat Psychol*. 2022;10(4):322–339 doi: 10.1037/lat0000212

10. Schnierle J, Christian-Brathwaite N, Louisias M. Implicit bias: what every pediatrician should know about the effect of bias on health and future directions. *Curr Probl Pediatr Adolesc Health Care*. 2019;49(2):34–44 PMID: 30738896 doi: 10.1016/j.cppeds.2019.01.003

11. Pachter LM, Coll CG. Racism and child health: a review of the literature and future directions. *J Dev Behav Pediatr*. 2009;30(3):255–263 PMID: 19525720 doi: 10.1097/DBP.0b013e3181a7ed5a

12. Alexander M. *The New Jim Crow: Mass Incarceration in the Age of Colorblindness*. New Press; 2020

13. Emergency Taskforce on Black Youth Suicide & Mental Health. *Ring the Alarm: The Crisis of Black Youth Suicide in America; A Report to Congress from the Congressional Black Caucus*. 2019. Accessed March 13, 2023. https://theactionalliance.org/resource/ring-alarm-crisis-black-youth-suicide-america

14. Galán CA, Meza JI, Ridenour TA, Shaw DS. Racial discrimination experienced by Black parents: enduring mental health consequences for adolescent youth. *J Am Acad Child Adolesc Psychiatry*. 2022;61(10):1251–1261 PMID: 35513191 doi: 10.1016/j.jaac.2022.04.015

15. Ben J, Cormack D, Harris R, Paradies Y. Racism and health service utilisation: a systematic review and meta-analysis. *PLoS One*. 2017;12(12):e0189900 PMID: 29253855 doi: 10.1371/journal.pone.0189900

16. Breland-Noble AM, Al-Mateen CS, Singh NN, eds. *Handbook of Mental Health in African American Youth*. Springer International Publishing; 2016 doi: 10.1007/978-3-319-25501-9

17. Weller BE, Harrison J, Adkison-Johnson C. Training a diverse workforce to address the opioid crisis. *Soc Work Ment Health*. 2021;19(6):568–582 doi: 10.1080/15332985.2021.1975014

18. Butler AM, Weller B, Titus C. Relationships of shared decision making with parental perceptions of child mental health functioning and care. *Adm Policy Ment Health*. 2015;42(6):767–774 PMID: 25577238 doi: 10.1007/s10488-014-0612-y

19. Anderson RE, Jones SCT, Navarro CC, McKenny MC, Mehta TJ, Stevenson HC. Addressing the mental health needs of Black American youth and families: a case study from the EMBRace intervention. *Int J Environ Res Public Health*. 2018;15(5):898 PMID: 29724068 doi: 10.3390/ijerph15050898

20. Osman A, Bagge CL, Gutierrez PM, Konick LC, Kopper BA, Barrios FX. The Suicidal Behaviors Questionnaire-Revised (SBQ-R): validation with clinical and nonclinical samples. *Assessment*. 2001;8(4):443–454 PMID: 11785588 doi: 10.1177/107319110100800409

21. Johnson JG, Harris ES, Spitzer RL, Williams JBW. The patient health questionnaire for adolescents: validation of an instrument for the assessment of mental disorders among adolescent primary care patients. *J Adolesc Health*. 2002;30(3):196–204 PMID: 11869927 doi: 10.1016/S1054-139X(01)00333-0

22. Craske M, Wittchen U, Bogels S, Stein M, Andrews G, Lebeu R. *Severity Measure for Generalized Anxiety Disorder—Child Age 11–17*. American Psychiatric Association; 2013

CHAPTER 13

Substance Use Policy and Practice

Hoover Adger Jr, MD, MPH, MBA, and J. Deanna Wilson, MD, MPH

Introduction

Substance use by youth (children, adolescents, and young adults) is a significant public health concern, with 1 in 5 adolescents reporting use of a substance in the past year. It affects all racial and ethnic groups across all socioeconomic classes. The proportion of high school seniors reporting any illicit drug use in their lifetimes declined from a peak of 55% in 1999 to a low of 47% in 2009, which remained relatively level through 2020. Marijuana remains the most common illicit drug used, with marked increases in youth vaping marijuana and nicotine in recent years. Alcohol remains the most common substance used. Although alcohol use has gradually declined across all grades, in 2020, 62% of high school seniors and 1 in 4 eighth graders still reported some experience with alcohol. About 14% of high school seniors also reported misusing prescription drugs.[1]

Youth are affected not only by their own substance use but also by familial substance use. Approximately 20 million individuals in the United States have a past-year history of substance use disorder (SUD), and many are parents or caregivers. More than 60% of pregnant women and people report using illegal substances, and 15% use them in a way that meets the criteria for SUD. These women and people are often younger and experience greater economic and social deprivation. Owing partially to its decriminalization, marijuana use during pregnancy has increased nearly 7-fold in the past decade. Similarly, the US opioid epidemic has led to a concomitant-use epidemic among pregnant women that has resulted in withdrawal syndromes in their prenatally exposed newborns. The long-term effects of early exposure to substances in utero are unknown.[2]

Approximately 8.7 million children are currently living with a parent/caregiver with SUD. Less than 10% of individuals with SUD receive treatment, a finding suggesting that many youth live with a parent/caregiver with an untreated disorder. Untreated SUD in parents/caregivers can lead to deterioration of family dynamics and deprivation of economic and social conditions, increasing the risk for adverse outcomes. Because historical approaches to SUD management have favored incarceration over treatment, particularly among racially minoritized populations, having SUD increases the likelihood of contact with the legal system, including the resulting impacts on youth development.[3] Children of parents/caregivers with SUD may lack consistency, stability, or emotional support owing to a chaotic family environment. Parental/caregiver substance use or SUD increases their risk of experiencing an unintentional injury, verbal abuse, or physical abuse. Parents and caregivers with SUD may demonstrate greater permissiveness, neglect, or under-socialization of their child, which is potentially devastating because it increases the likelihood of early initiation of substance use in their child.

Racial and Ethnic Disparities in Substance Use Prevention, Early Intervention, and Treatment

Although minoritized and other marginalized populations use substances at similar rates as white populations, minoritized populations are more likely to experience more severe consequences because of their use. Compared to their white counterparts, Black and Latine/x[a] populations experience greater mortality rates from substance use, greater severity of SUD, and increased vulnerability to legal system involvement.[4]

Racism is a normative experience for youth in minoritized populations in the United States. Black and Latine/x youth experience more significant barriers when accessing and completing substance use treatment, and fewer minoritized youth report satisfactory experiences within treatment programs than white youth.[5] These disparities are driven by intersectional racism, drug-related stigma, and associated discrimination. Structural racism is manifested in unequal enforcement of drug laws, lower access to evidence-based treatments, and greater odds of adverse substance-related health outcomes among minoritized populations.[6] Structural violence is expressed through stigma against people with SUD and through policies that disqualify people with SUD histories from access to public services, employment, education, and housing.[7]

Multiple studies show unacceptably low treatment rates for SUD among all adolescents, with Black and Latine/x adolescents experiencing the lowest treatment rates. For example, a cohort study of Medicaid-enrolled youth revealed that among those who experienced an opioid-related overdose, only 1 in 54 received treatment with evidence-based medications, with rates of treatment with medications among Black or Latine/x youth being less than 1%.[8] Disparities in treatment provision contribute to growing disparities in outcomes with the greatest escalation of opioid-related overdose deaths now seen among Black individuals in many localities.[9–11] Although much of the focus of the opioid epidemic has been on older adults, nearly 1 of every 10 deaths among youth aged 15 to 24 years now results from opioids.[12,13]

Transformation of Mental Health and Substance Use/SUD Service Delivery

The National Academy of Medicine, through its policy initiative 2021 Vital Directions for Health and Health Care, proposed 3 steps that are needed to address health professionals' current treatment deficits: transform the behavioral health system to meet youth where they are, decriminalize substance use to facilitate treatment and recovery, and raise awareness of social context and social needs as essential to effective care. It also advocates for a more diverse behavioral health workforce that can better understand the

---

[a] In this chapter, we use *Latine/x* when referring to people of Latin American origin or descent as a whole. It is a gender-neutral and gender-inclusive alternative to *Latino*. For a brief history of this term, including a rationale, refer to the book introduction.

social complexity of patients and their families. As pediatric health professionals, we must recognize the social complexity of substance use and SUD among youth and appreciate how intersectional racism and addiction-related stigma contribute to poor outcomes.

Addressing Racial and Ethnic Disparities in Substance Use/SUD Prevention and Treatment

Given the growing racial and ethnic diversity in the United States and the growing evidence of the association between racism and substance use outcomes among racially minoritized populations, pediatric health professionals must address the impact of racism and structural racism on their patients. First, we must facilitate a paradigm shift to integrate substance use/SUD prevention, early intervention, and treatment *as part of routine pediatric primary care*. To accomplish this, pediatric health professionals should improve early identification of substance use in the pediatric setting through implementation of validated screenings for substance use in adolescents and through nonjudgmental inquiry into substance use within families. Pediatric health professionals need to be familiar with evidence-based SUD treatment approaches and to be able to engage in conversations about substance use and SUD that are free of stigmatizing language while checking our own implicit and explicit biases.[14] Second, pediatric health professionals and programs should adopt an anti-racist strategy for substance use prevention, early intervention, and treatment. This will mean identifying specific social determinants of health and racial inequalities that affect minoritized youth and their families, understanding the way in which treatment programs and the medical system more broadly propagate structural racism and social disadvantage, and taking steps to mitigate this propagation within our own clinical practices or, more broadly, through advocacy.[15,16]

Patient-centered discussions on substance use require thoughtfully engaging youth and families to understand their values and how they weigh choices to make treatment decisions. These discussions can be complicated, particularly when patients and pediatric health professionals do not share the same cultural, racial, ethnic, or linguistic background, but they are vital. Unfortunately, attempts to address racial discordancy purely through cultural competency or diversity training will continue to fall short; we need to recruit and support a diverse and inclusive workforce that reflects the patients for whom we provide care.

Clinical, Policy, and Advocacy Approaches: A Path Forward

The low rates of SUD treatment among adolescents underscore a need for policies and interventions that improve screening, early intervention, and treatment efforts for all youth. Because minoritized youth remain at greater risk for more severe consequences from their substance use, we must identify ways to implement screening and treatment program referrals that prioritize equity and focus on the needs of Black and Latine/x youth. Because more than 90% of adolescents have a usual source of primary care, implementing short, validated screening instruments for substance use and SUD in primary care settings could help identify adolescents in need of treatment. Once adolescents with SUD have been identified, pediatric health professionals should work with them and their families to identify and refer for evidence-based treatment in the most appropriate setting. Particularly among those with opioid use disorder, we must prioritize access to evidence-based pharmacotherapy. Finally, we need more treatment programs that bridge residential neighborhoods and the community and are tailored to the developmental needs and social complexity of minoritized and other marginalized youth.

Summary

Substance use remains a common condition for youth from all racial and ethnic groups and all socioeconomic statuses. Although minoritized and other marginalized youth use substances at similar rates as white youth, minoritized youth are more likely to experience severe consequences and less likely to receive evidence-based treatment than their white counterparts. To address substance-use related disparities, pediatric health professionals need to integrate substance use/SUD prevention, early intervention, and treatment as part of routine pediatric primary care. To do so, we need to train a diverse workforce to engage in patient-centered conversations that are nonjudgmental, are compassionate, and acknowledge the impact of structural determinants of health, including racism, on substance use and treatment outcomes.

Recommendations

Following are specific, focused clinical, advocacy, and policy approaches that should be part of the path forward:

Patient- and Family-Directed

- Integrate routine screening for substance use and SUD within the pediatric primary care setting through evidence-based tools and skills that leverage youth strengths, such as motivational interviewing. Pediatric health professionals must receive ongoing training not only in how to recognize and treat substance use and SUD in primary care settings but also in how to recognize the role of their own implicit and explicit biases in treatment discussions.

Clinical Practice/Organizations/Systems

- Make it standard that treatment programs disseminate information on race and ethnicity, as well as outcome metrics, to better identify the programs most effective at addressing the needs of minoritized youth.

- Expand access to evidence-based interventions and therapies for youth, including state-of-the-art therapeutics and medications offered in specialty addiction treatment settings and in primary care settings serving youth.

Public Health Policy and Community Advocacy

- Develop treatment programs that are tailored to the developmental needs of youth and that address the impact of racial and other types of structural violence on well-being.

- Support positive youth development and behavioral models of care that respond to the unique circumstances of youth with SUD, and recognize the role that the direct effects of racism or discrimination may have on youth well-being. Moreover, gender nonconforming or gender minority youth experience disproportionately higher rates of substance use, homelessness, and suicidality. Pediatric health professionals need to recognize the impact of intersectional stigma and discrimination on youth outcomes and create treatment systems that are sensitive to these needs.

- Limit confrontation of minoritized and other marginalized youth with police. The default response for youth experiencing consequences from substance use should be a response from a trained substance use/SUD or mental health professional to de-escalate a crisis, should avoid unnecessary police contact, and should engage and direct the youth to the appropriate care.

References

1. Johnston LD, Miech RA, O'Malley PM, Bachman JG, Schulenberg JE, Patrick ME. *Monitoring the Future National Survey Results on Drug Use 1975–2021: Overview, Key Findings on Adolescent Drug Use.* Institute for Social Research, University of Michigan; 2022

2. Peterson BS, Rosen T, Dingman S, et al. Associations of maternal prenatal drug abuse with measures of newborn brain structure, tissue organization, and metabolite concentrations. *JAMA Pediatr.* 2020;174(9):831–842 PMID: 32539126 doi: 10.1001/jamapediatrics.2020.1622

3. Office of Juvenile Justice and Delinquency Prevention. Juvenile Residential Facility Census Databook. Accessed February 9, 2023. https://www.ojjdp.gov/ojstatbb/jrfcdb

4. Lau KSL, Rosenman MB, Wiehe SE, Tu W, Aalsma MC. Race/ethnicity, and behavioral health status: first arrest and outcomes in a large sample of juvenile offenders. *J Behav Health Serv Res.* 2018;45(2):237–251 PMID: 29238907 doi: 10.1007/s11414-017-9578-3

5. Goff PA, Jackson MC, Di Leone BAL, Culotta CM, DiTomasso NA. The essence of innocence: consequences of dehumanizing Black children. *J Pers Soc Psychol.* 2014;106(4):526–545 PMID: 24564373 doi: 10.1037/a0035663

6. Matsuzaka S, Knapp M. Anti-racism and substance use treatment: addiction does not discriminate, but do we? *J Ethn Subst Abuse.* 2020;19(4):567–593 PMID: 30642230 doi: 10.1080/15332640.2018.1548323

7. HealthyPeople.gov. Social determinants of health. Accessed February 9, 2023. https://www.healthypeople.gov/2020/topics-objectives/topic/social-determinants-of-health

8. Alinsky RH, Zima BT, Rodean J, et al. Receipt of addiction treatment after opioid overdose among Medicaid-enrolled adolescents and young adults. *JAMA Pediatr.* 2020;174(3):e195183 PMID: 31905233 doi: 10.1001/jamapediatrics.2019.5183

9. Furr-Holden D, Milam AJ, Wang L, Sadler R. African Americans now outpace whites in opioid-involved overdose deaths: a comparison of temporal trends from 1999 to 2018. *Addiction.* 2021;116(3):677–683 PMID: 32852864 doi: 10.1111/add.15233

10. Gomes T, Tadrous M, Mamdani MM, Paterson JM, Juurlink DN. The burden of opioid-related mortality in the United States. *JAMA Netw Open.* 2018;1(2):e180217 PMID: 30646062 doi: 10.1001/jamanetworkopen.2018.0217

11. Hall OT, Trimble C, Garcia S, Entrup P, Deaner M, Teater J. Unintentional drug overdose mortality in years of life lost among adolescents and young people in the US from 2015 to 2019. *JAMA Pediatr.* 2022;176(4):415–417 PMID: 35099529 doi: 10.1001/jamapediatrics.2021.6032

12. Marotta PL, Tolou-Shams M, Cunningham-Williams RM, Washington DM Sr, Voisin D. Racial and ethnic disparities, referral source and attrition from outpatient substance use disorder treatment among adolescents in the United States. *Youth Soc.* 2022;54(1):148–173 doi: 10.1177/0044118X20960635

13. Vidourek RA, King KA, Merianos AL, Bartsch LA. Predictors of illicit drug use among a national sample of adolescents. *J Subst Use.* 2018;23(1):1–6 doi: 10.1080/14659891.2017.1316782

14. Alinsky RH, Hadland SE, Quigley J, Patrick SW; American Academy of Pediatrics Committee on Substance Use and Prevention. Recommended terminology for substance use disorders in the care of children, adolescents, young adults, and families. *Pediatrics.* 2022;149(6):e2022057529 PMID: 35977095 doi: 10.1542/peds.2022-057529

15. Alegría M, Frank RG, Hansen HB, Sharfstein JM, Shim RS, Tierney M. Transforming mental health and addiction services. *Health Aff (Millwood).* 2021;40(2):226–234 PMID: 33476189 doi: 10.1377/hlthaff.2020.01472

16. Alegría M, Alvarez K, Ishikawa RZ, DiMarzio K, McPeck S. Removing obstacles to eliminating racial and ethnic disparities in behavioral health care. *Health Aff (Millwood).* 2016;35(6):991–999 PMID: 27269014 doi: 10.1377/hlthaff.2016.0029

Reproductive Justice–Informed Care for STIs, Contraception, and Abortion in Pediatrics

J'Mag Karbeah, PhD, MPH; Asha Hassan, MPH; and Rachel Hardeman, PhD, MPH

Introduction

As comprehensive contraceptive counseling has become the standard of care within pediatrics, new questions and concerns about patients' ages and abilities to make reproductive choices have arisen.[1] These concerns, which often reveal paternalistic beliefs toward adolescent fertility, can unintentionally lead to implicitly or explicitly coercive practices that harm youth (adolescents and young adults) and pose potential deterioration of the relationship they have with their pediatric health professional and future health professionals. In addition, pediatric health professionals working with patients from groups that have been racially and ethnically minoritized, subsequently referred to as *minoritized groups* for ease of reading, must consider how dominant racial narratives may influence their attitudes and recommendations.

Applying a reproductive justice lens is necessary to understand the complexity of pediatric reproductive and sexual health care for populations of color. This theoretical framework, developed in 1994 by Black women, seeks to reframe conversations about reproductive rights. Reproductive justice asserts that every person has "the human right to maintain bodily autonomy, have children, not have children, and parent the children they have in safe and sustainable communities."[2] In a more racially and gender-diverse generation than any generation before, it is essential to consider how embracing a framework can transform pediatric practice when this framework seeks to identify and eliminate various social and political systems that prevent all people from having reproductive freedom. The reproductive justice framework advocates for an asset-based approach to issues of sexuality and reproduction that can be effective and beneficial for youth across various racial, ethnic, and socioeconomic backgrounds.[3,4] For example, consistently incorporating positive development strategies that encourage youth to identify the skills and tools they already have to achieve their long-term goals in sexual and reproductive health visits reinforces that they possess the tools to succeed.

Pediatric health professionals are already skilled at embracing and advocating for the importance of bodily autonomy. The right to reproductive autonomy is perceived by many as a crucial part of one gaining full personhood.[3] Adopting a reproductive justice approach and interrogating the underlying and potentially racist narratives allow pediatric health professionals to extend their understanding of autonomy to sexual and reproductive health and to a broader set of patient issues.

The importance of centering the voices and experiences of youth with historically underrepresented racial,[4] gender, and sexual identities is critical when examining the significance of this framework in pediatric health care settings. In addition to championing this framework's call for bodily autonomy, pediatric health professionals must also acknowledge how experiences of racism and social disenfranchisement influenced creation of the reproductive justice framework and its application. This chapter highlights why racism has explicitly contributed to the histories of forced sterilization and reproductive coercion that made the reproductive justice framework necessary. It also highlights why it is crucial to center these histories in pediatric practice.

Pediatric Considerations

Acknowledging racism and the reproductive health inequities it creates is imperative to support the reproductive health of pediatric patients from minoritized groups. There is a dearth of studies that investigate racial differences in reproductive health care access, services, and adolescent outcomes. Patients who have been minoritized, including youth, are less likely to report contraceptive use but more likely to experience unwanted pregnancy and seek abortion care. These differences may be caused by issues with health care access, cultural norms and attitudes about contraception, and medical distrust from a legacy of institutional reproductive trauma.[5]

Youth navigating the reproductive health care system face unique challenges in achieving equitable care. The limited number of sites providing family planning counseling, as well as the provision, management, and removal services of contraceptive options specifically for youth, may compound racial inequities for pediatric populations.[6] Legal abortion restrictions and parental consent requirements hinder access for adolescents. Judicial bypass, required in many states for adolescents to access abortion care without parental consent, does not improve outcomes but increases the potential for harm by delaying necessary care. In addition, adolescent motherhood, linked to racial stereotypes, is often stigmatized in the health care setting.[7] Youth from minoritized groups are often treated as older than their developmental stages in our society; this *adultification* carries over into encounters with the reproductive health care system (refer to Chapter 31, Achieving Equity for Opportunity Youth). In American eugenics history, examples of the horrors of pediatric reproductive harm, including forced sterilization, exist.[8] More recently, minors in immigration detention centers faced significant restrictions in obtaining abortion care. Respecting the reproductive autonomy and decision-making of all adolescents is an ongoing concern in the American health care system.

Applying a Reproductive Justice Lens

Reproductive justice is a useful lens to assess equity within a wide range of reproductive health services, including contraception, abortion care, and sexually transmitted infection (STI) prevention and treatment (refer to Table 14–1 for additional information).

Table 14–1. Applying a Reproductive Justice Framework to Pediatric Health Care		
Reproductive Justice	**Current Limitations**	**Ways to Improve Practice**
Reproductive autonomy is a core tenet of the reproductive justice framework and is considered an inalienable right of all people.	Culturally held, often racialized beliefs and norms about sexuality, contraception, and reproduction both implicitly and explicitly influence pediatric health professionals. In clinical practice, decisions based on these cultural norms and narratives are often referred to as *biases* or *discrimination*.	Pediatric health professionals should center and be cognizant of historical and contemporary reproductive health injustices when developing patient-centered approaches.

Although providing informed choice in family planning is an essential element of reproductive autonomy, barriers manifest that may inhibit this. Health professional bias is the interpersonally manifested racist beliefs and narratives that are structurally and culturally embedded into care.[9] These narratives create and perpetuate norms about sexual activity, pregnancy, and parenthood that often villainize or pathologize individuals on the basis of age, marital status, race, and disability status.[5,9] Research indicates that these biases have a direct effect, with patients reporting that their choices are not always respected by health professionals, for example, when requesting to have long-acting reversible contraception devices removed.[10] The challenges of health professional bias are part of a long history of reproductive medical experimentation, eugenics policy, and forced sterilization in the United States that were directed at communities of color.[8,11]

Our history is always with us; however, health professionals must educate themselves on the many injustices that have affected reproductive health and the ensuing multigenerational consequences. They must apply a patient-centered approach to care. Historically, public health has relied on a risk-based strategy to frame reproductive health issues, focusing on "at-risk" groups and stigmatizing people of color. A risk-based strategy does not allow for the nuances of the complicated experience of unplanned pregnancy. Unlike disease or other outcomes assessed by health professionals, an unplanned pregnancy can be desired, unwanted, or met with ambivalence by pregnant women and people. Therefore, it is essential for health professionals not to pathologize unplanned pregnancies. Rethinking risk and applying a reproductive justice approach to public health policy strategy more firmly places health inequities into a social context. It also uplifts access to reproductive health services for all people as a human right.

The American Academy of Pediatrics recognizes the rights of adolescents to reproductive health care, including contraception and abortion. Beyond that, a renewed emphasis on structural and interpersonal factors such as racism and health professional bias is needed to educate and support health professionals caring for adolescents. Professionals must acknowledge the social determinants of health that predispose adolescents to these outcomes throughout the life course. Systemic inequities within society influence the quality of schools and the types of educational exposures for adolescents. Additionally, living in a racialized social system affects adolescent experiences with professionals in ways that may result in more bias and distrust that disincentivizes authentic and continued engagement with the health care system. Teenage pregnancy prevention efforts must focus on holistically supporting adolescents, without stigma.

With the rise in restrictions on abortion access, adolescents, particularly adolescents of color, deserve comprehensive and medically accurate reproductive health information, including options for abortion care, without fear of criminalization.[12] Pediatric health professionals can support their adolescent patients by equipping them with legal resources[13,14]; providing them with knowledge on how to identify and avoid pregnancy crisis centers, organizations known to give inaccurate and incomplete medical information[15]; and taking time to understand local financial support networks for abortion-seeking patients.[16]

Summary

It is important for pediatric health professionals, who often shape the relationships that individuals will have with the health care system throughout the life course, to understand how racism affects the reproductive and sexual health care experience of minoritized youth. The reproductive justice framework highlights why reproductive autonomy is essential for adolescents and emerging adults and aligns perfectly with the idea of bodily autonomy that pediatric health professionals already recognize. However, it is necessary to connect the need for bodily autonomy with understanding the impacts of historical and current racialized coercion, exploitation, and disenfranchisement on health care delivery. Pediatric health professionals must acknowledge and address the uncomfortable truth that implicitly and explicitly racist narratives exist within pediatric health care settings and that they can influence the access to and quality of care for minoritized youth seeking sexual and reproductive health services.

Recommendations

Patient- and Family-Directed

- Embrace positive youth development approaches that are specifically tailored for and by minoritized youth.

- Optimize individual pediatric competencies that include delivery of high-quality gynecologic services or a developmentally and age-appropriate referral source with a broad range of clinical skills delivered in a culturally proficient, patient-centered manner.
- Understand that abortion access is an adolescent health issue, and provide counseling and referral for all options to pregnant patients.
- Respect patient decisions about the use of short- and long-term contraceptives with the explicit understanding that an individual's ability to make their own reproductive decisions is a crucial part of their right to reproductive and bodily autonomy and development.

Clinical Practice/Organizations/Systems

- Explicitly name histories of gendered racism when discussing and adopting reproductive justice frameworks.
- Think critically about how explicit or implicit racialized narratives influence sexual and reproductive health recommendations/methods offered to adolescents with racial and ethnic identities, sexual orientations, and gender identities that have been minoritized.
- Challenge prevailing narratives on "at-risk" youth and teenage pregnancy, recognizing that these perspectives are often racialized.

Public Health Policy and Community Advocacy

- Advocate for policies and programs that ensure equitable access for all youth to resources that expand access to reproductive health care and therefore allow youth to thrive, including adequate funding for all schools, the expansion of medically accurate sex education programs, and the expansion of school-based health centers.

References

1. Cohen RE, Wilkinson TA, Staples-Horne M. The need for reproductive justice in pediatrics. *JAMA Pediatr.* 2021;175(12):1207–1208 PMID: 34542563 doi: 10.1001/jamapediatrics.2021.2978
2. Ross LJ. Understanding reproductive justice. In: McCann CR, Kim SK, Ergun E, eds. *Feminist Theory Reader: Local and Global Perspectives.* 5th ed. Routledge; 2021:77–82
3. Ross LJ, Solinger R. *Reproductive Justice: An Introduction.* University of California Press; 2017
4. Gilliam M. Youth reproductive justice: beyond choice, toward health equity. *Health Educ Behav.* 2020;47(4):640–641 PMID: 31893472 doi: 10.1177/1090198119876309
5. Troutman M, Rafique S, Plowden TC. Are higher unintended pregnancy rates among minorities a result of disparate access to contraception? *Contracept Reprod Med.* 2020;5(1):16 PMID: 33014415 doi: 10.1186/s40834-020-00118-5
6. Bell JM, Hartmann D. Diversity in everyday discourse: the cultural ambiguities and consequences of "happy talk". *Am Sociol Rev.* 2007;72(6):895–914 doi: 10.1177/000312240707200603
7. SmithBattle L. Walking on eggshells: an update on the stigmatizing of teen mothers. *MCN Am J Matern Child Nurs.* 2020;45(6):322–327 PMID: 32956170 doi: 10.1097/NMC.0000000000000655

8. Nathanson CA. *Dangerous Passage: The Social Control of Sexuality in Women's Adolescence.* Temple University Press; 1991

9. Johnson TJ. Intersection of bias, structural racism, and social determinants with health care inequities. *Pediatrics.* 2020;146(2):e2020003657 PMID: 32690807 doi: 10.1542/peds.2020-003657

10. Gilliam ML. Beyond coercion: let us grapple with bias. *Obstet Gynecol.* 2015;126(5):915–916 PMID: 26444119 doi: 10.1097/AOG.0000000000001116

11. Roberts D. *Killing the Black Body: Race, Reproduction, and the Meaning of Liberty.* Vintage Books; 1997

12. Bryson AE, Hassan A, Goldberg J, Moayedi G, Koyama A. Call to action: healthcare providers must speak up for adolescent abortion access. *J Adolesc Health.* 2022;70(2):189–191 PMID: 34916125 doi: 10.1016/j.jadohealth.2021.11.010

13. Judicial Bypass Wiki. Accessed February 9, 2023. https://judicialbypasswiki.ifwhenhow.org

14. Repro Legal Helpline. Abortion access: know your rights. Accessed February 9, 2023. https://www.reprolegalhelpline.org/sma-know-your-rights

15. Swartzendruber A, English A, Greenberg KB, et al. Crisis pregnancy centers in the United States: lack of adherence to medical and ethical practice standards; a joint position statement of the Society for Adolescent Health and Medicine and the North American Society for Pediatric and Adolescent Gynecology. *J Pediatr Adolesc Gynecol.* 2019;32(6):563–566 PMID: 31679958 doi: 10.1016/j.jpag.2019.10.008

16. National Network of Abortion Funds. Accessed February 9, 2023. https://abortionfunds.org

Part 2. Intersections of Racism and Health for Children and Adolescents

Section 2. Community Experiences of Racism

CHAPTER 15

The Role of Racism in Child and Adolescent Injuries

Benjamin D. Hoffman, MD

If a disease were killing our children at the rate unintentional injuries are, the public would be outraged and demand that this killer be stopped.

Former Surgeon General C. Everett Koop, MD, ScD

Introduction

Unintentional injuries kill more youth (children, adolescents, and emerging adults) in the United States than any other cause, with an average of more than 6,000 children and youth between the ages of 1 and 18 years dying annually (Figure 15–1). Over half these deaths have been associated with motor vehicles. Intentional injuries from firearms kill more than 2,000 additional children and youth annually through suicide and homicide, averaging approximately 870 child and 1,444 youth deaths.[1] Unfortunately, although pediatric health professionals have noted improvement in some areas, such as infant sleep-related death and motor-vehicle occupant fatalities, the injury epidemic persists.[2]

As with many epidemics, the risk is more significant for minoritized communities, often resulting from structural inequity and racism. Overall, American Indian/Alaska Native (AI/AN) and Black children experience the highest rates of intentional and unintentional injury–related deaths, approximately double the rate of white, non-Hispanic children[2] (Figure 15–2). Geographic location also plays a role, with youth in suburban and rural communities experiencing higher rates of motor-vehicle and drowning deaths.[3]

The Role of Inequity and Racism in Drowning

Drowning is the single leading cause of death for children aged 1 to 4 years and is a leading cause of unintentional injury–related death for males aged 15 to 19 years.[4] Risk factors and potential preventive interventions vary tremendously on the basis of age and geographic location. Most drownings occur in bathtubs among infants aged 0 to 1 year, often resulting from lapses in supervision. Black infants experience a 70% greater rate of bathtub drownings than white infants. Among 1- to 4-year-olds, over half of all drowning occurs in swimming pools. White children experience the highest rate of pool drowning, with a rate of 1.7 per 100,000, compared with 1.4 per 100,000 for Black toddlers and 1.2 per 100,000 for Hispanic toddlers.[5] This difference can be found partly

Figure 15–1. 10 Leading Causes of Death for US Children and Youth Aged 1 to 18 Years, With Relative Burden of Injury Mechanisms, Between 2010 and 2020

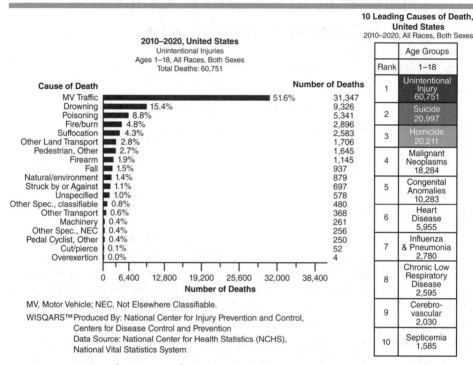

2010–2020, United States
Unintentional Injuries
Ages 1–18, All Races, Both Sexes
Total Deaths: 60,751

Cause of Death		Number of Deaths
MV Traffic	51.6%	31,347
Drowning	15.4%	9,326
Poisoning	8.8%	5,341
Fire/burn	4.8%	2,896
Suffocation	4.3%	2,583
Other Land Transport	2.8%	1,706
Pedestrian, Other	2.7%	1,645
Firearm	1.9%	1,145
Fall	1.5%	937
Natural/environment	1.4%	879
Struck by or Against	1.1%	697
Unspecified	1.0%	578
Other Spec., classifiable	0.8%	480
Other Transport	0.6%	368
Machinery	0.4%	261
Other Spec., NEC	0.4%	256
Pedal Cyclist, Other	0.4%	250
Cut/pierce	0.1%	52
Overexertion	0.0%	4

Number of Deaths (x-axis: 0, 6,400, 12,800, 19,200, 25,600, 32,000, 38,400)

MV, Motor Vehicle; NEC, Not Elsewhere Classifiable.

WISQARS™ Produced By: National Center for Injury Prevention and Control, Centers for Disease Control and Prevention
Data Source: National Center for Health Statistics (NCHS), National Vital Statistics System

10 Leading Causes of Death, United States
2010–2020, All Races, Both Sexes

Rank	Age Groups 1–18
1	Unintentional Injury 60,751
2	Suicide 20,997
3	Homicide 20,211
4	Malignant Neoplasms 18,284
5	Congenital Anomalies 10,283
6	Heart Disease 5,955
7	Influenza & Pneumonia 2,780
8	Chronic Low Respiratory Disease 2,595
9	Cerebro-vascular 2,030
10	Septicemia 1,585

Figure 15–2. Rates (per 100,000) of Injury Death for US Children and Youth Aged 1 to 18 Years by Race and Ethnicity Between 2010 and 2020

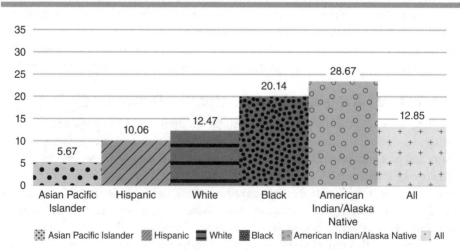

Asian Pacific Islander: 5.67
Hispanic: 10.06
White: 12.47
Black: 20.14
American Indian/Alaska Native: 28.67
All: 12.85

Legend: Asian Pacific Islander, Hispanic, White, Black, American Indian/Alaska Native, All

Data from Centers for Disease Control and Prevention. WISQARS Injury Data. Accessed February 10, 2023. https://www.cdc.gov/injury/wisqars/index.html.

because of circumstances related to socioeconomic factors: white children tend to drown in residential swimming pools, often inaccessible to children from minoritized communities. In contrast, Black and Hispanic children drown more often in public pools, most often at hotels and motels lacking lifeguards, and AI/AN children tend to drown most often in open water (eg, lakes, oceans).[4]

Considering protective factors for drowning, the development of water competence through swimming lessons is a cornerstone. In this context, the effects of systemic racism on drowning can be found. During our country's shameful institution of slavery, water often represented life and death as the medium for ships that were carrying people who had been enslaved. Although there was a proliferation of municipal swimming pools in the early 1900s, many established rules that prohibited entry to communities that had incomes below the federal poverty threshold and communities that had been minoritized, specifically Black people. Inequity in access to swimming skills training has amplified the drowning risk for children in families with limited incomes and for children of color.[6] Researchers at the University of Memphis have established that "there were significant racial differences concerning the fear of drowning, and adolescent African American females were notably more likely to fear drowning while swimming than any other group."[7] The rate of such fear-of-drowning responses by parents or caregivers of children from minoritized communities was also significantly different from their white counterparts'.[7] The same group of researchers has also shown that this fear manifests in Black and Latinx[a] children whose families have limited incomes and who lag behind their white counterparts in swimming ability.[8] Simply put, a legacy of racism dating back to the institution of slavery has directly led to increased drowning risk for Black children.

The Role of Racism in Land Management and Housing Policy

Systemic racism in the apportionment of land and housing has also disproportionately affected minoritized communities, leading to increased rates of injury.

The forcible removal of Indigenous populations from ancestral lands was a consistent strategy in the colonization of the United States, culminating in the Dawes Act of 1887. This act established Native American reservations and allowed the federal government to determine access to the resultant lands.[9] Often, this land was less desirable than the appropriated land, and poverty, associated with substandard infrastructure, including housing, roads, and access to health care, has adversely affected Indigenous communities. Consequently, AI/AN children have among the highest rates of injury-related death among all populations.[10] Refer to Chapter 7, Treaties, Public Health Service, and Health Status of Native American Children, Adolescents, and Young Adults.

---

[a] In this chapter, we use *Latinx* when referring to people of Latin American origin or descent as a whole. It is a gender-neutral and gender-inclusive alternative to *Latino*. For a brief history of this term, including a rationale, refer to the book introduction.

Black communities still experience tremendous negative effects from the historical practice of *redlining*, dating back to the 1930s. Redlining involved the stratification of neighborhoods by the Federal Housing Authority to mitigate risks to housing and mortgage lenders.[11] As a result, these communities experienced discriminatory disinvestment, adversely influencing the built environment, access to resources, and sociocultural structures that have resulted in worse health outcomes across several areas, including injury.[12-14] These effects manifest as increased firearm injury rates[15] and increased pedestrian injury rates,[16] among many others.

The Role of Child and Adolescent Health Advocates

Although the impacts of the racial disparities in injury are complex and manifold, pediatric health professionals can play a significant role in their mitigation as child and adolescent health advocates. *Physician advocacy* has been defined as "[a]ction by a physician to promote those social, economic, educational, and political changes that ameliorate the suffering and threats to human health and well-being that [they identify] through [their] professional work and expertise."[15] In that regard, we can think of 3 levels of physician advocacy engagement: individual advocacy, community advocacy, and policy and systems change advocacy.

Individual Advocacy

Anticipatory guidance and family-centered conversations are the centerpiece of health supervision care. *Bright Futures: Guidelines for Health Supervision of Infants, Children, and Adolescents* is the gold standard for pediatric primary care and includes specific guidance for every health supervision visit on age and developmentally germane injury prevention topics.[16] Pediatric health professionals are skilled in facilitating family-centered conversations, including tailored messaging around injury prevention. This should not solely be the domain of primary health professionals; rather, it should be integrated into subspecialty or inpatient care as circumstances warrant.

Families may need additional resources. Referrals for care coordination or social work can help them obtain resources in their community to help prevent injuries, including child passenger safety programs or hospital- or community-based injury prevention programs. Each of us can, and should, play a role in this advocacy at the individual child, adolescent, and family level. Although such advocacy is an essential tool and may help ensure that a particular family has resources, it is limited in changing a community's overall health and well-being.

Community Advocacy

Pediatric health professionals must also be able to work outside their traditional clinical roles and engage with governmental and community-based organizations to begin to address injury prevention at a greater systems level. The pioneering work of Barbara

Barlow and Danielle Laraque in developing the Harlem Hospital Injury Prevention Program is a sterling example. Through the development of coalitions with state and local governments, community-based organizations, schools, social service organizations, and families, they successfully worked to decrease injuries among children and youth in Harlem through community-based interventions, including playground development, bicycle-safety programs, arts and sports initiatives, and greening projects.[17]

Pediatric health professionals can lead similar initiatives or join existing ones, adding expertise and a trusted voice. It is essential that these efforts be family- and community-centered and that they foster authentic community engagement.[18] Community engagement can have a tremendous effect at the population level compared to the individual advocacy of clinical practice. Although pediatric training focuses on family-centered care and individual advocacy, the skills to effectively and authentically engage communities for advocacy are less consistently taught and learned. Further, the work of community advocacy is generally not explicitly considered part of a pediatric health professional's scope of work and is often completed during their unfunded time. Pediatric health professionals must be equipped with the knowledge and skills for this advocacy work, and we must push for funding through philanthropy, alternative payment methods, or community benefit dollars.

Policy and Systems Change Advocacy

Advocacy at the larger policy level, be it local, state, or federal, can have the greatest effect on decreasing the burden of child and adolescent injury. Child access prevention laws, which require safe storage of guns in homes, have reduced firearm-related deaths, including by homicide, suicide, and unintentional means.[19] Motor-vehicle occupant restraint laws, including for booster seats,[20] are similarly effective.

Pediatric health professionals are credible and trusted sources of expertise on issues affecting children, adolescents, and families. The ability to work with elected officials in developing and supporting policy intended to mitigate risks for injury can be a powerful tool. Although this process can be slow and frustrating, it can have a significant impact. Building relationships with institutional government-relations teams and partnering with professional organizations, such as the American Academy of Pediatrics and other pediatric associations, can be transformational. These entities have the resources and experience to help navigate the complicated landscape and provide guidance and support.

Summary

Inequity and systemic racism have exacerbated an already horrific epidemic of injury among children and adolescents. As Dr Koop noted, this epidemic receives relatively little attention compared to its impact on children, adolescents, families, and communities, with those from minoritized communities having borne a disproportionate burden for far too long.

Recommendations

Public Health Policy and Community Advocacy

To address the disparities in injury for minoritized communities, pediatric health professionals must

- Be both adept and effective in advocacy at the community and policy and systems change levels.

- Develop authentic relationships with families and communities, which are essential to effectively improve injury prevention for children and youth in a meaningful and culturally/linguistically appropriate manner.

- Implement evidence-based policy at all levels as one of the most effective means for decreasing injury risk.

  - Be able to develop and support policy interventions to mitigate risks for both intentional and unintentional injuries. Because so many of these risks are associated with social determinants of health, they cannot be adequately addressed in the course of our traditional clinical roles.

- Work to transform our practices to allow us to work outside that traditional clinical paradigm, both in the communities we serve and with those in power.

References

1. Centers for Disease Control and Prevention. Injury counts and rates. WISQARS Injury Data. Accessed February 10, 2023. https://wisqars.cdc.gov/reports

2. Pressley JC, Barlow B, Kendig T, Paneth-Pollak R. Twenty-year trends in fatal injuries to very young children: the persistence of racial disparities. *Pediatrics*. 2007;119(4):e875–e884 PMID: 17403830 doi: 10.1542/peds.2006-2412

3. Cunningham RM, Walton MA, Carter PM. The major causes of death in children and adolescents in the United States. *N Engl J Med*. 2018;379(25):2468–2475 PMID: 30575483 doi: 10.1056/NEJMsr1804754

4. Denny SA, Quan L, Gilchrist J, et al; American Academy of Pediatrics Council on Injury, Violence, and Poison Prevention. Prevention of drowning. *Pediatrics*. 2021;148(2):e2021052227 PMID: 34253571 doi: 10.1542/peds.2021-052227

5. Clemens T, Moreland B, Lee R. Persistent racial/ethnic disparities in fatal unintentional drowning rates among persons aged ≤29 years—United States, 1999–2019. *MMWR Morb Mortal Wkly Rep*. 2021;70(24):869–874 PMID: 34138831 doi: 10.15585/mmwr.mm7024a1

6. Bashir I. Teaching my Black son to swim. *New York Times*. June 15, 2001. Accessed February 10, 2023. https://www.nytimes.com/2021/06/15/well/family/black-children-swimming.html

7. Irwin CC, Irwin RL, Ryan TD, Drayer J. The legacy of fear: is fear impacting fatal and non-fatal drowning of African American children? *J Black Stud*. 2011;42(4):561–576 PMID: 21910272 doi: 10.1177/0021934710385549

8. Irwin CC, Irwin RL, Ryan TD, Drayer J. Urban minority youth swimming (in)ability in the United States and associated demographic characteristics: toward a drowning prevention plan. *Inj Prev*. 2009;15(4):234–239 PMID: 19651995 doi: 10.1136/ip.2008.020461

9. Gampa V, Bernard K, Oldani MJ. Racialization as a barrier to achieving health equity for Native Americans. *AMA J Ethics*. 2020;22(10):E874–E881 PMID: 33103650 doi: 10.1001/amajethics.2020.874

10. American Academy of Pediatrics Committee on Native American Child Health and Committee on Injury and Poison Prevention. The prevention of unintentional injury among American Indian and Alaska Native children: a subject review. *Pediatrics.* 1999;104(6):1397–1399 PMID: 10585996 doi: 10.1542/peds.104.6.1397

11. Rothstein R. *The Color of Law: A Forgotten History of How Our Government Segregated America.* Liveright; 2017

12. Lee EK, Donley G, Ciesielski TH, et al. Health outcomes in redlined versus non-redlined neighborhoods: a systematic review and meta-analysis. *Soc Sci Med.* 2022;294:114696 PMID: 34995988 doi: 10.1016/j.socscimed.2021.114696

13. Jacoby SF, Dong B, Beard JH, Wiebe DJ, Morrison CN. The enduring impact of historical and structural racism on urban violence in Philadelphia. *Soc Sci Med.* 2018;199:87–95 PMID: 28579093 doi: 10.1016/j.socscimed.2017.05.038

14. Coughenour C, Clark S, Singh A, Claw E, Abelar J, Huebner J. Examining racial bias as a potential factor in pedestrian crashes. *Accid Anal Prev.* 2017;98:96–100 PMID: 27716495 doi: 10.1016/j.aap.2016.09.031

15. Earnest MA, Wong SL, Federico SG. Perspective: physician advocacy: what is it and how do we do it? *Acad Med.* 2010;85(1):63–67 PMID: 20042825 doi: 10.1097/ACM.0b013e3181c40d40

16. American Academy of Pediatrics. Bright Futures. Accessed February 10, 2023. https://www.aap.org/en/practice-management/bright-futures

17. Laraque D, Barlow B, Durkin M, Heagarty M. Injury prevention in an urban setting: challenges and successes. *Bull N Y Acad Med.* 1995;72(1):16–30 PMID: 7581311

18. *Principles of Authentic Community Engagement.* Minnesota Dept of Health; 2018. Accessed February 10, 2023. https://www.health.state.mn.us/communities/practice/resources/phqitoolbox/docs/AuthenticPrinciplesCommEng.pdf

19. Azad HA, Monteaux MC, Rees CA, et al. Child access prevention firearm laws and firearm fatalities among children aged 0 to 14 years, 1991–2016. *JAMA Pediatr.* 2020;174(5):463–469 PMID: 32119063 doi: 10.1001/jamapediatrics.2019.6227

20. Mannix R, Fleegler E, Meehan WP III, et al. Booster seat laws and fatalities in children 4 to 7 years of age. *Pediatrics.* 2012;130(6):996–1002 PMID: 23129070 doi: 10.1542/peds.2012-1058

CHAPTER 16

The Impact of Racism on Education

Danielle G. Dooley, MD, Mphil; Desiree M. de la Torre, MPH, MBA;
Tonya Vidal Kinlow, MPA; and Gabrina L. Dixon, MD, MEd

You can't educate a child who isn't healthy, and you can't keep a
child healthy who isn't educated.
Joycelyn Elders, MD, Surgeon General of the United States,
1993–1994

Introduction

High-quality education is a critical factor for success in children and adolescents. Although all children and adolescents should have access to free public education, in the United States, communities of color have historically been denied equal access to quality education. Because of ongoing systemic racism, youth, including children, adolescents, and young adults, in the United States experience unequal educational opportunities depending on the schools they attend, the neighborhoods they live in, the color of their skin, and the financial resources of their families. Inequities are amplified when unanticipated events occur, such as the COVID-19 pandemic. Across the country, educational systems were initially unprepared to function in the presence of the highly infectious virus, which forced school closures, pushing learning into the virtual environment. Educators had to simultaneously build and implement virtual learning systems. The systemic disruption strained family environments, and youth bore the brunt of it. A study showed that by the end of the 2020–2021 school year, students were, on average, 5 months behind in math and 4 months behind in reading. For Black and Latino/a[a] students, this study noted that the losses in learning were more significant and therefore added to historical inequities in opportunity and achievement.[1] In addition, the COVID-19 pandemic affected children's social and emotional development.

Educational attainment is associated with longer life expectancy, better-paying jobs, and fewer health-harming behaviors.[2] Education is a critical pathway to financial security, stable employment, and social success. School is where children and adolescents go to learn and thrive and to become social actors. They spend a significant amount of time either attending school or working on school-related activities. Youth must be present and ready to learn to sufficiently leverage educational opportunities. Pediatric

---

[a] In this chapter, we use *Latino/a* when referring to people of Latin American origin or descent as a whole. It is a gender-neutral and gender-inclusive alternative to *Latino*. For a brief history of this term, including a rationale, refer to the book introduction.

health professionals and collaborators have a role in preparing children and adolescents to achieve this foundational standard. Education and health systems must partner to support successful growth and development of children, adolescents, and young adults. Although the country was unprepared to effectively respond to the pandemic at its outset, in the aftermath, it is incumbent that system leaders seize this opportunity for change to correct inequities and improve quality. Intentional partnerships between educators and health professionals can transform the well-being of children and adolescents and can help ameliorate the effects of racism on education.

Racism in the Educational Setting

Historical and systemic racism disproportionately disadvantage communities of color with respect to the educational experience. These practices include underfunding and under-resourcing of school districts serving large populations of students of color, both of which lead to inequities in access to quality facilities and teachers, advanced coursework, special education services, and high school graduation rates and chronic absenteeism rates. These inequities have an effect on educational attainment, which, in turn, can influence long-term health outcomes and contribute to further inequities in health. For example, on average, a person who graduated from college lives 9 years longer than someone who did not graduate from high school.[3] Therefore, pediatric health professionals should be aware of critical educational areas affected and shaped by racism at the interpersonal and systemic levels, including stereotype threat, school discipline, early childhood education, standardized testing, multilingual learner supports, and extracurricular opportunities.

Stereotype Threat and Its Impact on Academic Performance for Youth of Color

Stereotype threat is "being at risk of confirming, as self-characteristic, a negative stereotype about one's group."[4] Stereotype threat can lead to disengaged learning and lower academic performance.[5] For example, medical students of races and ethnicities that are underrepresented in medicine (URiM) noted facing lower expectations of achievement during their secondary schooling because of their race and ethnicity, affecting their journey to medical school. They felt as though educators expected less of them during their education.[6] To be protected from this threat, children and adolescents need to learn in an anti-racist environment.

School Discipline

There are well-documented disproportionate rates of school suspensions and expulsions for children of color in the educational setting. The National Center for Education Statistics found that Black students (13.7%) and American Indian/Alaska Native students (6.7%) experienced more out-of-school suspensions than white peers (3.4%).[7]

The Civil Rights Project at the University of California, Los Angeles, found that Black students lost 103 days per 100 students enrolled because of out-of-school suspensions, as compared to 21 days for their white peers. Disparities are magnified when gender is also examined, with Black girls experiencing 77 days of lost instruction per 100 students enrolled because of out-of-school suspensions, which was 7 times the rate of their white female peers.[8] Research shows that a major contributor to these disparities is inequitable disciplinary practices, with differential treatment of Black and white children and adolescents within the same school for the same infraction.[9]

Early Childhood Education

Access to high-quality early childhood education (ECE) improves school readiness for children, and "for young children living in poverty, [it] contribute[s] to their intellectual and social development in childhood and their school success, economic performance, and reduced commission of a crime in adulthood."[10] However, inequities exist in access to quality ECE. For example, few states offer universal preschool. In addition, the infrastructure challenges combined with tuition charges; complex mechanisms for benefits eligibility to offset the costs; waiting lists; low wages for early childhood teachers, particularly teachers of color; and lack of access to evening and weekend care for families who have nontraditional work schedules result in disparate access to high-quality ECE.[11]

Standardized Testing

The No Child Left Behind Act of 2001 was intended to address inequities in academic achievement and to hold states more accountable for educational quality. A component of the act is mandatory standardized testing in schools.[12] The original purpose of standardized testing was to evaluate teachers to ensure that students were learning. It has also been used to rank students' performances and help determine educational funding levels for schools and districts. However, these tests are known to be biased against children of color, through reinforcement of stereotype threat and a cultural bias in content geared toward white test takers whose families have high incomes.[13,14] A multifactorial evaluation system (eg, student portfolios and interpersonal skills) should be used when evaluating students rather than one standard of measurement via testing.

Multilingual Learner Supports

Approximately 10% of public school students are multilingual learners in the United States, with 75% of those identifying Spanish as their native language.[15] Although the US Supreme Court affirmed that school districts receiving federal funding must provide access to linguistic support for children learning English, the quality and availability of that support vary widely across the country. Inconsistent linguistic support widens the opportunity gap between students learning English and students speaking English proficiently. In addition, there are inequities in access to and enrollment in ECE programs, advanced coursework, and dual-credit programs for multilingual learners.[16]

Extracurricular Activities, Gifted and Talented Programs, and Pathway Programs

Participation in extracurricular activities is associated with positive youth development outcomes (refer to Chapter 26, Positive Youth Development as an Anti-racist Strategy), including improved academic performance and lower risk-taking behaviors, such as lower rates of substance use. However, there are disparities in access to extracurricular activities, with Latino/a youth experiencing the least participation in sports and non-sports. The rate of participation among Black youth in non-sports extracurricular activities as compared to the rate among white youth has widened over time, reflecting structural inequities in access to programming.[17] Black students in the third grade are one-half as likely as their white peers to be included in gifted programs in public schools.[18,19] Structural inequities in access to extracurricular activities; gifted and talented programs; and pathway programs contribute to disparities in educational experiences and outcomes for students. Pathway programs can help diversify the health care workforce and eliminate health care disparities. Physicians of races and ethnicities that are URiM are more likely to care for under-resourced populations.[20] Pathway programs, such as a medical student–run program with hands-on experience for children and adolescents from backgrounds that are URiM, can expose youth at a young age to careers in medicine.[21]

Summary

Pediatric health teams and institutions can address the effects of racism in the education system by becoming school friendly. A School-Friendly Health System (SFHS) is a health system actively working to ensure all children and adolescents achieve optimal health and reach their full academic potential. The SFHS framework contains 5 core principles that reflect a broad range of competencies, practices, and policy positions that health care experts and community partners view as characteristic of an SFHS (Table 16–1).[22] The table below provides recommendations for application of the SFHS principles at the patient, practice, and policy levels. As students, educators, parents, caregivers, and pediatric health professionals face the ongoing challenges of racial inequities, it is critical for the health and education sectors to partner to address the needs of children and adolescents.

Recommendations

Table 16–1. School-Friendly Health System Framework			
School-Friendly Health System Principle	**Patient- and Family-Directed**	**Clinical Practice/ Organizations/ Systems**	**Public Health Policy and Community Advocacy**
1. AWARENESS School-Friendly Health Systems are familiar with and responsive to the culture, policies, and needs of the school systems and student populations they serve.	● Ask questions about patients' school experiences and racism. Be alert to responses that could indicate potential health or social challenges. Patient interactions must be grounded in deep cultural competency enhanced through the lens of cultural humility. ● Ask about stressors at school (eg, bullying and cyberbullying based on race)[a] and social determinants of health often associated with racism (eg, neighborhood safety, poverty, housing inequity, and academic access) to connect families to resources.[b–d]	● Embrace a philosophy of co-design and co-implementation for all programming and use a racial equity lens. ● Pediatric health professionals leading school-based interventions/ school programs should collaborate with school system leaders and staff to address racism at school.	● Advocate for policies promoting racial equity in the education sector and the broader community. ● Advocate for implicit bias training of school personnel. ● Advocate that the quality of education in segregated urban, suburban, and rural communities be designed better to optimize vocational attainment and educational milestones for all students.

(continued on next page)

Table 16–1 (*continued*)			
School-Friendly Health System Principle	**Patient- and Family-Directed**	**Clinical Practice/ Organizations/ Systems**	**Public Health Policy and Community Advocacy**
2. ALIGNMENT School-Friendly Health Systems have a cohesive strategy for collaborating with schools and communities that aligns with those partners' needs and goals.	● Reinforce health- and academic-supporting messages. ● Identify the impacts of racism and the educationally relevant health disparities in the community, and apply this understanding to patient interactions.	● Refer to the American Academy of Pediatrics Council on School Health materials on ways that pediatric health professionals can get involved with and support schools.[e]	● View academic initiatives (eg, reading, tutoring, and extracurricular activities) as health-promoting/ social justice initiatives and within the health care mission to support. ● Advocate for educational programs, such as Head Start and early childhood education access.
3. ACCESSIBILITY School-Friendly Health Systems make themselves accessible to school partners and collaborate with those partners to optimize students' learning experience.	● Strive for greater communication with parents, caregivers, and families and with schools and school personnel.	● Support a curriculum of social justice programming in a school or school district. ● Provide support for school-based health centers and school nursing, especially for under-resourced schools.	● Advocate for mental health services, school-based health centers, and school nursing in schools.

Table 16–1 (*continued*)			
School–Friendly Health System Principle	**Patient- and Family-Directed**	**Clinical Practice/ Organizations/ Systems**	**Public Health Policy and Community Advocacy**
4. ACCOUNTABILITY School-Friendly Health Systems set organizational goals that support children's learning and set metrics and incentives that reinforce those priorities.	● Implement training in pediatric residency programs and for practicing pediatric health professionals that addresses school health and educates professionals on how to address racism in education.	● Incorporate metrics and incentives in clinical care to address educational attainment. ● Implement systems to ensure that all patients and families know they are welcome, they will be treated with mutual respect, and they will receive high-quality care through the tenets of family- and patient-centered care.[f]	● Advocate for the collection of data in the district or community that identifies educational disparities and inequities.
5. FAMILY ENGAGEMENT School-Friendly Health Systems collaborate and share power with families, understanding that they are the most important conduits between health systems and schools.	● Communicate effectively with parents, caregivers, and families about their children's health, education, and experiences with racism. Work with families to bolster racial identities. ● Help families navigate barriers that could be preventing their children from attending school.	● Recognize that parents, caregivers, and families bring their own experiences with racism and education and identify programming and resources to support them.	● Advocate for resources for families that support school attendance and engagement. ● Advocate for resources that support multilingual learners and their families.

[a] Brown P, Tierney C. Media role in violence and the dynamics of bullying. *Pediatr Rev.* 2011;32(10):453–454.
[b] American Academy of Pediatrics Council on Community Pediatrics. Poverty and child health in the United States. *Pediatrics.* 2016;137(4):e20160339.

[c] Slopen N, Shonkoff JP, Albert MA, et al. Racial disparities in child adversity in the U.S.: interactions with family immigration history and income. *Am J Prev Med.* 2016;50(1):47–56.

[d] Sampson RJ, Wilson WJ. Toward a theory of race, crime, and urban inequality. In: Hagan J, Peterson RD, eds. *Crime and Inequality.* Stanford University Press; 1995:56.

[e] American Academy of Pediatrics Council on School Health. American Academy of Pediatrics. Accessed February 10, 2023. https://www.aap.org/en/community/aap-councils/council-on-school-health.

[f] American Academy of Pediatrics Committee on Hospital Care, Institute for Patient- and Family-Centered Care. Patient- and family-centered care and the pediatrician's role. *Pediatrics.* 2012;129(2):394–404.

References

1. Dorn E, Hancock B, Sarakatsannis J, Viruleg E. COVID-19 and education: the lingering effects of unfinished learning. McKinsey & Company. July 27, 2021. Accessed February 10, 2023. https://www.mckinsey.com/industries/education/our-insights/covid-19-and-education-the-lingering-effects-of-unfinished-learning

2. Allison MA, Attisha E, Lerner M, et al; American Academy of Pediatrics Council on School Health. The link between school attendance and good health. *Pediatrics.* 2019;143(2):e20183648 PMID: 30835245 doi: 10.1542/peds.2018-3648

3. Robert Wood Johnson Foundation. *The Relationship Between School Attendance and Health.* Robert Wood Johnson Foundation; 2022. Accessed March 28, 2023. https://files.eric.ed.gov/fulltext/ED592870.pdf

4. Steele CM, Aronson J. Stereotype threat and the intellectual test performance of African Americans. *J Pers Soc Psychol.* 1995;69(5):797–811 PMID: 7473032 doi: 10.1037/0022-3514.69.5.797

5. Shelvin KH, Rivadeneyra R, Zimmerman C. Stereotype threat in African American children: the role of Black identity and stereotype awareness. *Rev Int Psychol Soc.* 2014;27(3–4):175–204

6. Dixon G, Kind T, Wright J, Stewart N, Sims A, Barber A. Factors that influence underrepresented in medicine (UIM) medical students to pursue a career in academic pediatrics. *J Natl Med Assoc.* 2021;113(1):95–101 PMID: 32771220 doi: 10.1016/j.jnma.2020.07.014

7. The National Center for Education Statistics. Status and trends in the education of racial and ethnic groups. Accessed February 10, 2023. https://nces.ed.gov/programs/raceindicators/highlights.asp

8. Losen DJ, Martinez P. *Lost Opportunities: How Disparate School Discipline Continues to Drive Differences in the Opportunity to Learn.* University of California, Los Angeles, The Civil Rights Project; 2020. Accessed February 10, 2023. https://www.civilrightsproject.ucla.edu/research/k-12-education/school-discipline/lost-opportunities-how-disparate-school-discipline-continues-to-drive-differences-in-the-opportunity-to-learn/Lost-Opportunities_EXECUTIVE-SUMMARY_v17.pdf

9. Ryberg R, Her S, Temkin Cahill D, Harper K. Despite reductions since 2011–12, Black students and students with disabilities remain more likely to experience suspension. Black Children and Families. ChildTrends. August 9, 2021. Accessed April 5, 2023. https://www.childtrends.org/publications/despite-reductions-black-students-and-students-with-disabilities-remain-more-likely-to-experience-suspension

10. Schweinhart LJ, Montie J, Xiang Z, Barnett WS, Belfield CR, Nores M. *The High/Scope Perry Preschool Study Through Age 40: Summary, Conclusions, and Frequently Asked Questions.* High/Scope Press; 2005. Accessed February 10, 2023. https://nieer.org/wp-content/uploads/2014/09/specialsummary_rev2011_02_2.pdf

11. Johnson-Staub C. *Equity Starts Early: Addressing Racial Inequities in Child Care and Early Education Policy.* Center for Law and Social Policy; 2018. Accessed February 10, 2023. https://www.clasp.org/wp-content/uploads/2022/01/Equity-Starts-Early-Executive-Summary.pdf

12. No Child Left Behind Act. HR 1, 107th Congress (2001). Accessed February 10, 2023. https://www.congress.gov/bill/107th-congress/house-bill/1

13. Couch MII, Frost M, Santiago J, Hilton A. Rethinking standardized testing from an access, equity and achievement perspective: has anything changed for African American students? *J Res Initiat.* 2021;5(3). Accessed February 10, 2023. https://digitalcommons.uncfsu.edu/jri/vol5/iss3/6

14. Marmol E. The undemocratic effects and underlying racism of standardized testing in the United States. *Crit Intersect Educ.* 2016;4:1–9. Accessed February 10, 2023. https://jps.library.utoronto.ca/index.php/cie/article/view/26430

15. National Center for Education Statistics. English learners in public schools. In: *The Condition of Education 2022.* Institute of Education Sciences, US Dept of Education; 2022:chap2. Accessed February 10, 2023. https://nces.ed.gov/programs/coe/indicator/cgf

16. US Department of Education. Educational experiences of English language learners. Accessed February 10, 2023. https://www2.ed.gov/datastory/el-experiences/index.html

17. Meier A, Hartmann BS, Larson R. A quarter century of participation in school-based extracurricular activities: inequalities by race, class, gender and age? *J Youth Adolesc.* 2018;47(6):1299–1316 PMID: 29536328 doi: 10.1007/s10964-018-0838-1

18. Grissom JA, Redding C. Discretion and disproportionality: explaining the underrepresentation of high-achieving students of color in gifted programs. *AERA Open.* 2016;2(1): doi: 10.1177/2332858415622175

19. Dynarski S. Why talented Black and Hispanic students can go undiscovered. *New York Times.* April 8, 2016. Accessed February 10, 2023. https://www.nytimes.com/2016/04/10/upshot/why-talented-black-and-hispanic-students-can-go-undiscovered.html

20. Marrast LM, Zallman L, Woolhandler S, Bor DH, McCormick D. Minority physicians' role in the care of underserved patients: diversifying the physician workforce may be key in addressing health disparities. *JAMA Intern Med.* 2014;174(2):289–291 PMID: 24378807 doi: 10.1001/jamainternmed.2013.12756

21. Muppala VR, Janwadkar RS, Rootes A, Prakash N. Creating a pipeline for minority physicians: medical-student-led programming. *Cureus.* 2021;13(4):e14384 PMID: 33987050 doi: 10.7759/cureus.14384

22. Children's National. School-Friendly Health System framework FAQs. Accessed February 10, 2023. https://childrensnational.org/advocacy-and-outreach/child-health-advocacy-institute/community-affairs/school-partnerships/school-friendly-health-system-framework-faqs

The Impact of Interactions With Law Enforcement on the Health of Racially Minoritized Youth

Monique Jindal, MD, MPH, and Alexandra M. S. Corley, MD, MPH

It made me realize how dangerous it is to be Black in America.... We shouldn't have to walk on eggshells around police officers, the same people that are supposed to protect and serve. We are looked at as thugs, animals, and criminals, all because of the color of our skin.

Darnella Frazier, an 18-year-old witness who filmed the murder of George Floyd[1]

Introduction

Groups that have been racially minoritized, subsequently referred to as *minoritized groups* for ease of reading, have long experienced disproportionate violence at the hands of law enforcement and other policing bodies. There has been heightened awareness of this in recent years because the emergence of police body-camera footage and social media have brought police-mediated harassment, violence, and death into our living rooms. Children and adolescents are not exempt from interactions with the police because they may be secondarily exposed to law enforcement through their caregivers, passively surveilled within their neighborhoods, and even directly subjected to contact with border patrol agents, school resource officers, and community police. Pediatric health professionals should understand the historical and present-day contexts of police interactions and their impact on child health and well-being.

Historical Context

Policing on American soil predates the US Constitution. The earliest police forces were patrols that existed to monitor the movement of Black people, both enslaved and freed, and worked to uphold the institution of slavery, through terrorism, violence, and oppression.[2] With that as a foundation, structural racism in policing has manifested in historical and contemporary times: just a generation ago, police were responsible for enforcing racist policies, such as the black codes, which incarcerated Black people who could not prove their employment status on demand. Such policies were replaced by disproportionate drug sentencing in the 1970s and 1980s and policing strategies such as "stop and frisk" in the 1990s, which continue today and disproportionately affect communities of color. This historical context provides the background for the continual use of policing to maintain social order through a racial hierarchy, ultimately perpetuating injustices for systemically oppressed groups.

Law Enforcement Contact

Today, law enforcement contact can be both direct and indirect. Contact with law enforcement may or may not be preceded by a crime or infraction and may or may not conclude in arrest or detainment. For example, 75% of young Black men were more likely than white men to be accosted by police in New York City yet were less likely to have contraband. Pediatric health professionals should broaden their definition of contact with law enforcement and work to decouple "delinquency" from police interaction.[3]

Direct Contact

Nearly 30 million people had contact with the police in 2018, with young adults aged 18 to 24 years experiencing the most police contact.[4] Although we often think of direct police-initiated contact via stops or arrests in public spaces or vehicles, youth (child, adolescent, and young adult) engagement with law enforcement might also occur in specialized settings such as schools. School resource officers are sworn law enforcement officials employed in elementary, middle, or high schools by the local or federal government and having the power to detain and arrest students. They are present in as many as 68% of schools.[5] There are approximately 14 million students in schools that have school resource officers but do not have a counselor, nurse, social worker, or psychologist. As a result, schools with police on-site are 3.5 times more likely to have student arrests than schools without police on-site, with students from Black, Latinx,[a] Native American, Pacific Islander, and Native Hawaiian communities and students with disabilities bearing the brunt of this practice.[6] Children and adolescents may also interact with law enforcement during travel into or out of the country.

Indirect Contact

Children also interface with police indirectly, from undergoing community and school surveillance to witnessing their caregivers' and neighbors' experiences. A youth's caregivers or neighbors may be involved with law enforcement via stops by law enforcement, arrests, jail, or prison sentences or while on parole. More than 5 million youth have a caregiver who has been incarcerated. Research demonstrates that these youth have worse health and well-being outcomes.[7] An incarcerated parent/caregiver or family member may create a social void for individual children, families, and communities. Improving technology and the increased use of social media have also allowed youth to witness secondhand police violence, which can similarly affect health and well-being.[8]

---

[a] In this chapter, we use *Latinx* when referring to people of Latin American origin or descent as a whole. It is a gender-neutral and gender-inclusive alternative to *Latino*. For a brief history of this term, including a rationale, refer to the book introduction.

Conceptual Frameworks Linking Police Contact and Health

Youth contact with police is recognized as an adverse childhood experience (ACE), which can harm development. (Refer to Chapter 24, Racial Trauma and Trauma-Informed Practice, for a detailed description of the impact of ACEs.)

Even beyond the age of 20 years, youth have reduced ability for impulse control and future orientation, which can lead to risk-taking behaviors, susceptibility to negative peer influence, and reduced capacity for decision-making in highly charged situations. These facets of youth development disproportionately expose youth to poor interactions with police.

Although contact with police can be understood through the lens of ACEs and youth development, it has also been recognized as an exceptional form of trauma because of the following unique circumstances:

- Violence from police is state sanctioned.
- Police are pervasive and unavoidable.
- There are limited options for recourse.
- Organizational culture deters internal accountability.
- Interactions reinforce a racial order.
- Contact is stigmatizing.
- There are high stakes owing to officers being armed.
- Police contact challenges conventional beliefs regarding safety.[9]

Impact on Health and Well-being

In 2021, more than 1,000 people were shot and killed by the police in the United States,[10] with the risk of being killed by the police being highest among Black men. Although death is the most severe consequence, there is a growing body of literature demonstrating the less obvious effects of police contact on pediatric and adolescent health in several domains: mental health; risk behaviors; physical health; exposure to emotional, physical, and sexual abuse; academic outcomes; and a youth's relationship with society.

Mental Health

Pediatric research reveals that police contact is associated with psychological distress, anger, externalizing behaviors, fear, posttraumatic stress and anxiety, depression,[11] and self-harm.[12] The literature on adults has shown associations with psychotic experiences[13] and suicidal ideation.[14]

Risk Behaviors

Police contact is also associated with substance use and sexual risk behaviors. Some suggest that being over-policed leads to a sense of alienation from society that affects a youth's future orientation and, ultimately, their willingness to take risks.[11]

Physical Health

Pediatric physical health outcomes are understudied. However, one study shows that expectant mothers who experience discrimination by police tend to have infants with low birth weights,[15] and adolescents who experience contact with police tend to rate their overall self-reported health as poor[16] and to experience sleep deprivation.[17] Literature about adults has shown relationships with diabetes, high blood pressure, asthma,[18] and increased waist circumference.[19]

Exposure to Emotional, Physical, and Sexual Abuse

Youth report exposure to multiple forms of abuse by police, including racial slurs and other demeaning language, such as "stupid." Youth also experience emotional abuse, including being abandoned in unknown neighborhoods far from home or being forced to walk home without shoes. Reported physical abuse includes being punched, kicked, and choked. Last, youth, especially females, report sexual assault by officers.[11]

Academic Outcomes

Funding for police in schools is associated with decreased high school graduation and college enrollment.[20] Relatedly, adolescents who experience arrest are twice as likely to drop out of school and to obtain 1 to 2 fewer years of education.[21] Children living in highly policed areas have lower standardized test scores and grade point averages.[22,23]

A Youth's Relationship With Society

Police contact predisposes youth to further police contact through a mechanism known as *labeling*. After youth are arrested once, they are 7.5 times as likely to be arrested again regardless of criminal involvement.[24] Interactions with police and the youth legal system are also experiences of racial socialization, in which a youth gains an understanding of their place in society, such as the development of increased feelings of diminished self-worth or more resignation to injustice when compared with others.[11] Last, interactions with police are associated with less involvement with other institutions, such as health care, education, and the labor market.[25,26]

Summary

Police contact is a critical determinant of health. Wide racial disparities persist in police contact, resulting in health inequities, including death, for people from minoritized groups. Children, adolescents, and their families live in this reality, and those from minoritized groups may be at risk for worse health and well-being outcomes because of disproportionate police contact. Pediatric and adolescent health professionals should be well versed in policing as a potential source of trauma for children, adolescents, and their families and should advocate for evidence-based interventions that reduce exposure to police contact.

Recommendations

Patient- and Family-Directed

- Provide space for children to discuss their experiences with police with trusted individuals.
- Provide anticipatory guidance.
- Support legislation that ensures youth-specific limits to police contact.

Clinical Practice/Organizations/Systems

- Advocate for developmentally appropriate, interdisciplinary, and trauma-informed approaches to law enforcement within institutions and communities.
- Screen youth and their families for hyper-surveillance in their communities and direct or vicarious contact with police.
- Screen youth for the symptoms associated with police contact, such as anger, fear, stress, depression, and difficulties in school.
- Provide referrals for mental health services and individualized education programs as needed.
- Collect standardized data on police harm that prioritizes pediatric populations.
- Educate medical students, residents, and faculty on the health impacts of police contact, particularly among communities of color; on the health impacts of experiences of racism; and on trauma-informed care.

Public Health Policy and Community Advocacy

- Create youth-specific guidelines for stops, citations, and arrests (eg, ending youth arrest for minor possession of marijuana, as implemented in Philadelphia; setting youth-specific limits to use of touch, force, and speech).
- Remove police from youth-serving institutions (eg, clinics, hospitals, schools).
- Partner with school administrators to minimize punitive contact with police.
- Form interdisciplinary collaborations with community outreach workers, social workers, or mental health professionals to ensure the presence of authority with youth-specific and trauma-informed care training during youth-police interactions.
- Advocate for comprehensive police training on trauma-informed care, youth development, ACEs, implicit bias, and racism.

- Support reallocation of resources from law enforcement to social services, housing, health care, and education.
- Encourage use of body cameras and civilian-oversight boards.

References

1. Hernandez J. Read this powerful statement from Darnella Frazier, who filmed George Floyd's murder. NPR. May 26, 2021. Accessed February 13, 2023. https://www.npr.org/2021/05/26/1000475344/read-this-powerful-statement-from-darnella-frazier-who-filmed-george-floyds-murd

2. Hadden SE. *Slave Patrols: Law and Violence in Virginia and the Carolinas.* Harvard University Press; 2001 doi: 10.2307/j.ctv1g809mv

3. Weaver VM, Papachristos A, Zanger-Tishler M. The great decoupling: the disconnection between criminal offending and experience of arrest across two cohorts. *RSF.* 2019;5(1):89–123 doi: 10.7758/rsf.2019.5.1.05

4. Harrell E, Davis E. *Contacts Between Police and the Public, 2018 – Statistical Tables.* Bureau of Justice Statistics; 2020. NCJ publication 255730

5. Javdani S. Policing education: an empirical review of the challenges and impact of the work of school police officers. *Am J Community Psychol.* 2019;63(3–4):253–269 PMID: 30729533 doi: 10.1002/ajcp.12306

6. Whitaker A, Torres-Gullién S, Morton M, et al. *Cops and No Counselors: How the Lack of School Mental Health Staff Is Harming Students.* American Civil Liberties Union; 2019

7. Wildeman C, Goldman AW, Turney K. Parental incarceration and child health in the United States. *Epidemiol Rev.* 2018;40(1):146–156 PMID: 29635444 doi: 10.1093/epirev/mxx013

8. Campbell F, Valera P. "The only thing new is the cameras": a study of US college students' perceptions of police violence on social media. *J Black Stud.* 2020;51(7):654–670 doi: 10.1177/0021934720935600

9. DeVylder J, Fedina L, Link B. Impact of police violence on mental health: a theoretical framework. *Am J Public Health.* 2020;110(11):1704–1710 PMID: 32941068 doi: 10.2105/AJPH.2020.305874

10. 1,110 people have been shot and killed by police in the past 12 months. *Washington Post.* January 5, 2023. Accessed February 13, 2023. https://www.washingtonpost.com/graphics/investigations/police-shootings-database

11. Jindal M, Mistry KB, Trent M, McRae A, Thornton RLJ. Police exposures and the health and well-being of Black youth in the US: a systematic review. *JAMA Pediatr.* 2022;176(1):78–88 PMID: 34491292 doi: 10.1001/jamapediatrics.2021.2929

12. Jackson DB, Testa A, Fix RL, Mendelson T. Adolescent police stops, self-harm, and attempted suicide: findings from the UK millennium cohort study, 2012–2019. *Am J Public Health.* 2021;111(10):1885–1893 PMID: 34554817 doi: 10.2105/AJPH.2021.306434

13. DeVylder JE, Cogburn C, Oh HY, et al. Psychotic experiences in the context of police victimization: data from the survey of police-public encounters. *Schizophr Bull.* 2017;43(5):993–1001 PMID: 28369639 doi: 10.1093/schbul/sbx038

14. DeVylder JE, Frey JJ, Cogburn CD, et al. Elevated prevalence of suicide attempts among victims of police violence in the USA. *J Urban Health.* 2017;94(5):629–636 PMID: 28534243 doi: 10.1007/s11524-017-0160-3

15. Collins JW Jr, David RJ, Symons R, Handler A, Wall S, Andes S. African-American mothers' perception of their residential environment, stressful life events, and very low birthweight. *Epidemiology.* 1998;9(3):286–289 PMID: 9583420 doi: 10.1097/00001648-199805000-00012

16. McFarland MJ, Geller A, McFarland C. Police contact and health among urban adolescents: the role of perceived injustice. *Soc Sci Med.* 2019;238:112487 PMID: 31445303 doi: 10.1016/j.socscimed.2019.112487

17. Testa A, Jackson DB, Semenza D. Unfair police treatment and sleep problems among a national sample of adults. *J Sleep Res.* 2021;30(6):e13353 PMID: 33870581 doi: 10.1111/jsr.13353

18. Sewell AA, Jefferson KA. Collateral damage: the health effects of invasive police encounters in New York City. *J Urban Health*. 2016;93(suppl 1):42–67 PMID: 26780583 doi: 10.1007/s11524-015-0016-7

19. McFarland MJ, Taylor J, McFarland CAS. Weighed down by discriminatory policing: perceived unfair treatment and Black-white disparities in waist circumference. *SSM Popul Health*. 2018;5:210–217 PMID: 30094316 doi: 10.1016/j.ssmph.2018.07.002

20. Weisburst EK. Patrolling public schools: the impact of funding for school police on student discipline and long-term education outcomes. *J Policy Anal Manage*. 2019;38(2):338–365 doi: 10.1002/pam.22116

21. Kirk DS, Sampson RJ. Juvenile arrest and collateral educational damage in the transition to adulthood. *Sociol Educ*. 2013;88(1):36–62 PMID: 25309003 doi: 10.1177/0038040712448862

22. Legewie J, Fagan J. Aggressive policing and the educational performance of minority youth. *Am Sociol Rev*. 2019;84(2):220–247 doi: 10.1177/0003122419826020

23. Ang D. The effects of police violence on inner-city students. *Q J Econ*. 2020;136(1):115–168 doi: 10.1093/qje/qjaa027

24. Liberman AM, Kirk DS, Kim K. Labeling effects of first juvenile arrests: secondary deviance and secondary sanctioning. *Criminology*. 2014;52(3):345–370 doi: 10.1111/1745-9125.12039

25. Brayne S. Surveillance and system avoidance: criminal justice contact and institutional attachment. *Am Sociol Rev*. 2014;79(3):367–391 doi: 10.1177/0003122414530398

26. Alang S, McAlpine DD, Hardeman R. Police brutality and mistrust in medical institutions. *J Racial Ethn Health Disparities*. 2020;7(4):760–768 PMID: 31989532 doi: 10.1007/s40615-020-00706-w

CHAPTER 18

Youth Legal System

Mikah Owen, MD, MPH, MBA, and Stephenie Wallace, MD, MSPH

Introduction to the Youth Legal System in the United States

The youth legal system (commonly referred to as the *juvenile justice system*) in the United States is a complex, decentralized system that is largely administered at the state and local levels.[1] As a result, youth (child, adolescent, and young adult) legal system policies, patterns, and trends vary. Despite the regional variations, the general structure and processes of the youth legal system are similar across jurisdictions. Working knowledge regarding the design and process of the youth legal system can help inform clinical and advocacy efforts intended to improve outcomes and eliminate racial and ethnic disparities for youth involved in the legal system. Figure 18–1 illustrates the typical progression of delinquency cases through the youth legal system.

Over the past 2 decades, the United States has seen steady declines in youth arrest (decreasing 58% from 2010 to 2019),[2] detention (decreasing 54% from 2005 to 2019),[3] and residential placement rates (decreasing 65%, in a 1-day census count of youth in residential placement from 1997–2019).[4] However, despite these steady declines, there remain significant racial and ethnic disparities throughout the youth legal system.

Racial and Ethnic Disparities Within the Youth Legal System

As detailed in Table 18–1, racial and ethnic disparities exist at virtually every decision point within the youth legal system, from arrest to residential placement. Theories regarding the cause of these disparities are commonly grouped into 2 broad, conceptual frameworks: *differential treatment* and *differential offending.*[5-7]

The differential treatment hypothesis postulates the disparities result from racial bias across the youth legal system.[5-7] In support of this hypothesis, multiple studies have demonstrated bias against youth of color at all decision points within the legal system. For example, the authors of a 2018 review article examined official processing data at various justice system decision points from 2001 to 2014 and found that 79% of studies showed that being a person of color had some disadvantageous effect on youth processed in the legal system.[8]

Conversely, the differential offending hypothesis attributes racial and ethnic disparities within the youth legal system to differences in the frequency and severity of delinquent behavior or criminal acts by youth of color.[5-7] This hypothesis does not ascribe

Figure 18-1. Typical Progression of Delinquency Cases Through the US Juvenile Justice System

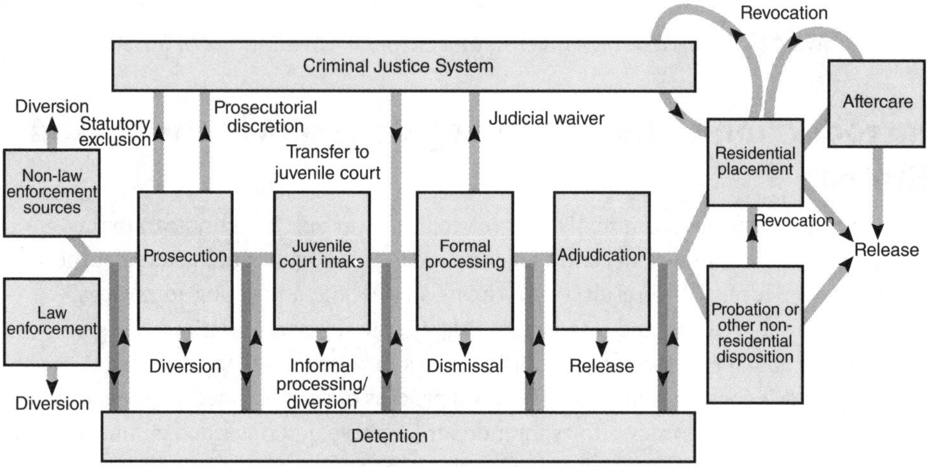

Reproduced from Office of Juvenile Justice and Delinquency Prevention. Juvenile justice system structure and process: case flow diagram. Statistical Briefing Book. Accessed February 13, 2023. https://www.ojjdp.gov/ojstatbb/structure_process/case.html.

Table 18-1. 2019 Data on Racial and Ethnic Disparities in the US Juvenile Justice System

Relative Rate	White	Minority	Black	Hispanic	American Indian/ Alaska Native	Asian/ Pacific Islander
Juvenile arrest[a]	—	1.8	2.4	Not reported	1.5	0.3
Cases referred to juvenile court[b]	—	1.5	2.9	1.0	1.2	0.2
Cases diverted out of the youth legal system[b]	—	0.7	0.6	0.8	0.8	0.9
Juvenile detainment (youth held in a detention facility before adjudication)[b]	—	1.5	1.4	1.6	1.2	1.3

Table 18–1 (*continued*)						
Relative Rate	**White**	**Minority**	**Black**	**Hispanic**	**American Indian/ Alaska Native**	**Asian/ Pacific Islander**
Cases adjudicated as delinquent (youth found guilty)[b]	—	1.0	0.9	1.1	1.1	1.0
Adjudicated cases resulting in secure confinement[b]	—	1.4	1.4	1.4	1.1	1.0
Cases judicially waived to criminal (adult) court[b]	—	1.3	1.5	0.9	0.8	0.9
Juvenile residential placement[c]	—	2.3	4.4	1.3	3.3	0.3

— indicates that the ratio of rates compares the rates of each minority group to white youth.
[a] Office of Juvenile Justice and Delinquency Prevention. Statistical Briefing Book. Released June 24, 2022. Accessed February 13, 2023. https://www.ojjdp.gov/ojstatbb/special_topics/qa11502.asp?qaDate=2020&text=yes.
[b] Office of Juvenile Justice and Delinquency Prevention. Statistical Briefing Book. Released January 10, 2023. Accessed March 23, 2023. https://www.ojjdp.gov/ojstatbb/special_topics/qa11602.asp?qaDate=2020&text=yes.
[c] Office of Juvenile Justice and Delinquency Prevention. Statistical Briefing Book. Released May 21, 2021. Accessed February 13, 2023. https://www.ojjdp.gov/ojstatbb/special_topics/qa11801.asp?qaDate=2019&text=yes.

differences in delinquent behavior to biological or genetic differences between races or ethnicities. Instead, it posits that youth of color are more likely to experience a variety of risk factors for delinquency (eg, poverty, harsh discipline practices in schools, exposure to violence, incarceration of a parent or caregiver, toxic stress) and are thus more likely to have delinquent behavior or commit criminal acts. Much of the research supporting this hypothesis relies on official records, such as rates of arrests, confinements, and convictions. When empirical data are cited from official records, which are influenced by inequities in legal system practices (eg, over-policing of historically disenfranchised neighborhoods, racial profiling of youth of color), it may overestimate the differences in delinquent behavior and criminal acts between racial and ethnic groups and therefore perpetuate bias within the literature.

Although helpful as conceptual frameworks, the differential treatment and differential offending hypotheses represent an oversimplification of the causes of racial and ethnic disparities within the youth legal system. These disparities exist within the broader context of racial and ethnic disparities in child health and well-being. Collectively, they are rooted in inequities in the social and environmental determinants of health and in the failure of public policies to address these inequities adequately.

Federal and State Efforts to Reduce Racial and Ethnic Disparities Within the Youth Legal System

The Juvenile Justice Delinquency and Prevention Act was first enacted in 1974. In 2018, it was reauthorized by the Juvenile Justice Reform Act and now requires states to "implement policy, practice, and system improvement strategies…to identify and reduce racial and ethnic disparities among youth who come into contact with the juvenile justice system."[9] The reauthorization act also requires that states[9]

- Establish coordinating bodies composed of juvenile justice stakeholders to advise efforts to reduce racial and ethnic disparities.

- Identify and analyze data on race and ethnicity at decision points in juvenile justice systems to determine which points create racial and ethnic disparities.

- Develop and implement an action plan to reduce racial and ethnic disparities within local juvenile justice systems.

States that do not comply with these guidelines may lose up to 20% of their annual federal grant allocation.[9]

The Role of Pediatric Health Professionals in Improving Outcomes and Eliminating Racial and Ethnic Disparities Within the Youth Legal System

As trusted youth advocates, pediatric health professionals have a critical role in preventing youth delinquency, improving outcomes for youth involved in the legal system, and eliminating racial and ethnic disparities within the youth legal system. Pediatric health professionals and others can realize this role through the provision of clinical care and participation in advocacy activities to reform the youth legal system and address the root causes of juvenile delinquency.

Clinical Care

Opportunities for clinical intervention for youth involved, or at risk of being involved, in the legal system extend beyond the walls of juvenile detention facilities. In the community setting, pediatric health professionals can leverage the medical home to promote primary, secondary, and tertiary prevention efforts to prevent delinquency and improve outcomes for youth with current or past involvement in the legal system. To achieve this objective, pediatric health professionals should be aware of risk factors for youth delinquency and the high prevalence of medical, mental health, developmental, social, and legal needs of youth involved in the legal system. There is no single risk factor that can predict the likelihood that a child or an adolescent will engage in delinquent behavior. Instead, "the effect is cumulative: the more risk factors present in a youth's life, the greater the probability of the youth [having] delinquent [behavior]."[10]

A literature review by the Office of Juvenile Justice and Delinquency Prevention showed that risk factors for youth delinquency are commonly grouped into 5 domains: individual, peer, family, school, and community. Relevant risk factors may include, but are not limited to, poverty, family conflict, low-performing schools, harsh discipline policies in schools, increased police presence in communities, exposure to significant childhood adversity and toxic stress, and incarceration of a parent/caregiver.[10,11] When considering risk factors, pediatric health professionals should recognize how racism and discrimination may lead to increased prevalence of delinquency risk factors among youth of color. Pediatric health professionals can enhance primary, secondary, and tertiary prevention efforts by monitoring for key risk factors, providing (or coordinating) comprehensive medical and mental health care, and maintaining linkages to community-based organizations that can help address the unique needs of youth involved in the legal system and their families.

For youth held in confinement, pediatric health professionals can help ensure that they have access to the same levels and standards of medical, mental health, and oral care as youth not held in confinement. To help achieve this, pediatric health professionals can encourage juvenile detention facilities to adopt and comply with the National Commission on Correctional Health Care *Standards for Health Services in Juvenile Detention and Confinement Facilities.*[12] Pediatric health professionals can also help maintain continuity of care by connecting youth with a medical home before release from the confinement facility.

Summary

As experts in the medical and developmental needs of children and adolescents, pediatric health professionals represent natural advocates for a youth legal system that is developmentally appropriate and is free of racial and ethnic biases. Advocates can work to bring awareness and dismantle inequities in all settings, especially the legal system, so the negative consequences are not compounded in the lives of our youth. However, many pediatric health professionals may struggle to understand their role in advocating for structural changes to the youth legal system. The American Academy of Pediatrics policy statement "Advocacy and Collaborative Health Care for Youth Involved in the Justice System"[11] highlights priority goals for juvenile justice/legal reform for pediatric health professionals and others interested in engaging in juvenile justice/legal advocacy activities. Additionally, pediatric health professionals can work with the American Academy of Pediatrics chapter in their states, justice/legal-involved youth and their families, state and local government organizations, and community organizations serving justice/legal-involved youth to identify priority opportunities for youth legal system reform in their local jurisdictions.

Regarding eliminating racial and ethnic disparities within the juvenile system, these disparities must be considered within the broader context of disparities in child health and well-being. This book highlights the pervasive nature of racism and discrimination and discusses the many ways in which racism and discrimination contribute to the inequities referenced in this chapter. This book also offers opportunities for pediatric health professionals to respond to mitigate the effects of racism and achieve health equity. Taken together, the strategies discussed in this book offer a road map for mitigating the effects of racism and reducing racial and ethnic disparities within the youth legal system and beyond.

Recommendations

Clinical Practice/Organizations/Systems

- Promote primary, secondary, and tertiary prevention efforts to prevent delinquency and improve outcomes for youth with current or past involvement in the legal system.
- Monitor for key risk factors, provide (or coordinate) comprehensive medical and mental health care, and maintain linkages to community-based organizations that can help address the unique needs of youth involved in the legal system and their families.

Public Health Policy and Community Advocacy

- Support research and advocacy efforts intended to eliminate racial and ethnic disparities within the legal system. Research and advocacy efforts should include an examination of racial and/or ethnic bias throughout the legal system.
- Collaborate with federal, state, and local government organizations and with organizations serving youth involved in the legal system, as well as affected youth, parents, and caregivers, to mitigate the impact of interpersonal and structural racism.

References

1. National Research Council, Institute of Medicine. *Juvenile Crime, Juvenile Justice.* National Academies Press; 2001 doi: 10.17226/9747
2. Office of Juvenile Justice and Delinquency Prevention. Statistical Briefing Book. Released November 16, 2020. Accessed February 13, 2023. https://www.ojjdp.gov/ojstatbb/crime/qa05101.asp?qaDate=2019
3. Office of Juvenile Justice and Delinquency Prevention. Statistical Briefing Book. Released June 22, 2021. Accessed February 13, 2023. https://www.ojjdp.gov/ojstatbb/court/qa06301.asp?qaDate=2019
4. Office of Juvenile Justice and Delinquency Prevention. Statistical Briefing Book. Released May 21, 2021. Accessed February 13, 2023. https://www.ojjdp.gov/ojstatbb/corrections/qa08201.asp?qaDate=2019
5. Developmental Services Group Inc. *Disproportionate Minority Contact (DMC).* Office of Juvenile Justice and Delinquency Prevention; 2014. Accessed February 13, 2023. https://ojjdp.ojp.gov/sites/g/files/xyckuh176/files/media/document/disproportionate_minority_contact.pdf
6. National Research Council Division of Behavioral and Social Sciences Education Committee on Assessing Juvenile Justice Reform and Committee on Law and Justice. *Reforming Juvenile Justice: A Developmental Approach.* Bonnie R, Johnson RL, Chemers BM, Schuck JA, eds. National Academies Press; 2013
7. Kakade M, Duarte CS, Liu X, et al. Adolescent substance use and other illegal behaviors and racial disparities in criminal justice system involvement: findings from a US national survey. *Am J Public Health.* 2012;102(7):1307–1310 PMID: 22594721 doi: 10.2105/AJPH.2012.300699

8. Spinney E, Cohen M, Feyerherm W, Stephenson R, Yeide M, Shreve T. Disproportionate minority contact in the U.S. juvenile justice system: a review of the DMC literature, 2001 to 2014, II. *J Crime Justice*. 2018;41(5):596–626 doi: 10.1080/0735648X.2018.1516156

9. Juvenile Justice Reform Act. HR 6964, 115th Congress (2018). Accessed February 13, 2023. https://www.congress.gov/bill/115th-congress/house-bill/6964/text

10. Development Services Group Inc. *Risk Factors for Delinquency*. Office of Juvenile Justice and Delinquency Prevention; 2015. Accessed February 13, 2023. https://ojjdp.ojp.gov/sites/g/files/xyckuh176/files/media/document/risk_factors.pdf

11. Owen MC, Wallace SB; American Academy of Pediatrics Committee on Adolescence. Advocacy and collaborative health care for youth involved in the justice system. *Pediatrics*. 2020;146(1):e20201755 PMID: 32376728 doi: 10.1542/peds.2020-1755

12. National Commission on Correctional Health Care. *Standards for Health Services in Juvenile Detention and Confinement Facilities*. National Commission on Correctional Health Care; 2015

CHAPTER 19

Environmental Justice

Jerome A. Paulson, MD, and Bethany L. Carlos, MD, MPH

Environmental [j]ustice…is the fair treatment and meaningful involvement of all people regardless of race, color, national origin, or income with respect to the development, implementation and enforcement of environmental laws, regulations and policies…. [It] will be achieved when everyone enjoys: [t]he same degree of protection from environmental and health hazards, and [e]qual access to the decision-making process to have a healthy environment in which to live, learn, and work.

US Environmental Protection Agency[1]

Introduction: Environmental (In)Justice

You practice in your hometown. The once-thriving city had included a prominent Black middle-class business community. In the early 1950s, the government built a highway that divided the neighborhood. This change brought truck, bus, and automobile traffic, resulting in reduced community cohesion and neglect by the city government over time. The mother of your patient has lived in this neighborhood all her life, including during her pregnancies. She had a preterm newborn with complications from cerebral palsy and cognitive delay. Her second child was born at 35 weeks' gestation with a low birth weight. At the 2-month visit, she asks about the prognosis for that child.

Your rural practice serves children from migrant families. Aside from limited continuity of care caused by frequent relocation, you are concerned about their temporary housing, which is next to fields that have been sprayed with different products 2 to 3 times since they moved there. The caregivers in the family are Spanish speaking and cannot read the warning labels on the pesticides they use. The children are at risk for neurocognitive delay and other problems caused by exposure to pesticides.

You practice at a medical center owned and operated by a Native nation and located on a reservation. Although the reservation has existed for more than 100 years, the US government has not yet invested in adequate water infrastructure. Because of this, the family does not have access to clean, reliable water sources for drinking and basic sanitation. You have treated their young children for multiple gastrointestinal, respiratory, and skin infections.

These are examples of environmental injustice affecting pediatric health professionals and the patients, families, and communities in which they practice. Environmental problems, such as climate change, exposure to lead, indoor and outdoor air pollution, pesticides, and other toxic chemicals, are more likely to affect communities that have been minoritized, communities with low or very low incomes, or communities that have limited proficiency in English.

Discussion of environmental issues may feel different or uncomfortable for the pediatric health professional and the patient or parent/caregiver. However, evidence shows that parents are receptive to discussing climate change in clinical settings.[2] Therefore, today's pediatric health teams must be familiar with a range of issues related to environmental justice.[3] Some of the most important topics follow.

Common Environmental Health Issues in Pediatrics

Climate Change

Climate change is the most important problem confronting humanity and affects health. As fossil fuel use grows, the atmosphere traps heat, worsening heat waves, raising sea levels, and causing storms, more frequent/severe wildfires, more extreme precipitation events/flooding, and worsening drought. These changes influence physical health, mental health, infectious disease patterns, and food and water insecurity. For example, the increased number of wildfires that are associated with climate change can cause physical injury and worsen air pollution. Patients experience stress associated with displacement from fires and anxiety about future fires. The worsening air pollution leads to respiratory illnesses, especially for those with chronic respiratory diseases. The increasing burden of climate change further strains communities that are already resource limited.[4,5]

Indoor and Outdoor Air Pollution

Air pollutants are composed of ozone, particulate matter, carbon monoxide, nitrogen dioxide, and sulfur dioxide. There can also be indoor air pollutants adding further exposures to developing children, contributing to more asthma and allergy symptoms in affected children and adolescents.

Communities facing environmental injustice are more likely to experience higher levels of air pollutants caused by proximity to roads and industries.[6–8]

Clean Water

Contaminants include infectious organisms, fecal matter, inorganic chemicals, or organic compounds.[9] Communities with public water sources are regulated through policies such as the Clean Water Act and the Safe Drinking Water Act. Private well owners are responsible for testing their water.

Millions of people are without access to quality drinking water. Some communities in the United States still do not have indoor plumbing. On Native American reservations, 48% of households do not have running water. Native American people are 19 times more likely to live in a home without indoor plumbing/running water than white people.[10] This number is increasing as more water infrastructure deteriorates without funding allocated for replacement. Large swaths of Appalachia also do not have indoor plumbing. Many cities have water pipes made of lead that need to be replaced.[11] Also, placing large-scale infrastructure projects, such as methane pipelines, can put drinking water at risk.

Toxic Waste Sites, Landfills, and Incinerators

Communities with limited resources and communities of color are more likely to live near a toxic waste site, a landfill, or an incinerator.[12] Today's landfills must meet stringent design, operation, and closure requirements that were established under the Resource Conservation and Recovery Act. Unfortunately, many older landfills do not meet modern standards, and newer landfills may contaminate communities despite standards.

Transportation

Transportation infrastructure includes systems to move people safely, including highways, roads, trains, and buses. Transportation equity ensures fair access to reliable, safe, and affordable solutions, including bicycle lanes and sidewalks. In the United States, 45% of families do not have access to public transit.[13]

Individuals in limited-income, minoritized communities that are already facing environmental injustice are less likely to own vehicles.[14] Rural communities with even fewer public transportation solutions must rely on private vehicles. Urban communities have more public transportation stops in higher-income communities, leaving the workers who need public transportation the most with more cumbersome and lengthy commutes.

Quality Housing as Part of the Built Environment

Ideally, all children and adolescents should reside in homes that provide adequate shelter for each individual, including protection against weather, harmful exposures, and criminal activity. This includes the building material and the surrounding built environment. Unfortunately, members of environmental justice communities are more likely to live in homes with poor ventilation, inefficient energy, lead, carbon monoxide, and degrading built materials.

Environmental justice communities have built environments with less green space, fewer sidewalks, higher crime rates, and closer proximities to toxic waste sites. Zoning and discriminatory structural practices have been implicated in forcefully removing children and families from long-term housing. The lingering effects of redlining, or the historical practice of preventing individuals from limited-income and minoritized communities from obtaining mortgages, continue to affect the environmental health of communities. For example, formerly redlined areas now have a disproportionate amount of concrete and asphalt. Therefore, those areas are hotter and are referred to as *urban heat islands.*[15]

Although gentrification leads to the transformation of neighborhoods from low value to high value, these changes may have the unintended (or perhaps intended) consequences of displacing long-term residents and businesses caused by higher rents, mortgages, and property taxes.

Exposure to Lead

Lead is a neurotoxin that is detrimental to health at all ages. The primary route of exposure is oral. The exposure can be in the form of lead in paint (large, visible particles or dust) in the child's residence, lead in water from lead pipes, or lead-containing solder used to join pipes together. Lead in water can occur in homes or schools.

Limited-income, minoritized communities are more likely to reside in *older home stock,* meaning a higher risk of old lead paint.[16] The presence of lead in water can be determined only by testing, and when lead is found, the only complete solution is excavation and replacement of all piping. Lead pipes occur in many communities irrespective of economic status or race.

Management of Environmental Issues

Unfortunately, many communities already experience the harmful effects of environmental injustice. Pediatric health professionals have an opportunity in clinical practice to counsel patients, parents, and caregivers.

Managing environmental justice problems is not something that a pediatric health professional and a patient or parent/caregiver can usually achieve on their own. Sustainable changes occur outside of clinical walls.

The involvement of community organizations should be sought out. Access to legal resources can sometimes be helpful or even be essential. There are more than 450 sites in the country in which health professionals and lawyers come together in medicolegal partnerships.[17] Accessing a medicolegal partnership can be useful in trying to manage the housing problems of individual patients. Moreover, long-term advocacy with politicians and corporations is necessary if a whole community is exposed to high levels of air or water pollution or a toxic waste site.

Health professionals can play a supportive role in community organizations by providing technical expertise on health matters. Pediatric health professional input is welcomed in the policy space. Pediatric health professionals can connect with a local group to champion environmental justice issues facing the communities they serve. Local policy makers can be reached by phone, electronically, or in person to meet with constituents and other interested parties to advance policy to protect children and families.

Summary

Examples of environmental (in)justice abound in the United States and around the globe. This long history and the current practices of systemic racism have significant health impacts. Pediatric health professionals have the expertise to be part of groups that tackle these problems.

Recommendations

Table 19–1 provides suggestions on how to implement recommendations made in this chapter.

Table 19–1. Putting Environmental Justice Into Practice		
Topic	**Patient- and Family-Directed**	**Clinical Practice/Organizations/Systems and Public Health Policy and Community Advocacy**

Recommendations relevant to all topics	● Encourage patients and families to join with others in the community who are concerned about the same health hazard. These may include
	  • Local, grassroots organizations
	  • Traditional environmental organizations (eg, League of Conservation Voters)
	  • Faith organizations
		● Empower your patients and their families to become voices for the injustices that are burdening their communities. Particularly, adolescents can be a powerful voice when advocating.
		● If you are concerned about environmental justice issues in a community but are unsure of the community's needs, become an advocate by bringing together community leaders to conduct a community needs assessment.
		● Pediatric Environmental Health Specialty Units (www.pehsu.net) can be consulted on any of the topics mentioned in this table.

(continued on next page)

Table 19–1 (continued)		
Topic	**Patient- and Family-Directed**	**Clinical Practice/Organizations/Systems and Public Health Policy and Community Advocacy**
Climate change	● Ensure that families recognize that climate solutions are health solutions. ● Encourage families to • Consume more plant-based meals and reduce meat consumption. • Increase time spent outdoors. • Use active transportation such as walking, biking, and public transportation as much as possible.	● Use the American Board of Pediatrics Maintenance of Certification module on climate, health, and equity.[18]
Indoor and outdoor air pollution	● Periodically assess your area's daily air-quality index on AirNow (www.airnow.gov) and teach your caregivers, parents, and patients to check this index regularly. ● Encourage families to wear face coverings, minimize time outside, and shift to indoor play and physical activity on days with poorer air quality. ● Discourage smoking indoors, and support smoking cessation among adults and adolescents who smoke in the home. ● If cost-effective, support switching from wood- or methane gas–burning energy sources to electric heating and cooking to reduce indoor pollutants.	● Work with community members to establish an Air Quality Flag program in their neighborhood.[19]

Table 19–1 (*continued*)		
Topic	**Patient- and Family-Directed**	**Clinical Practice/Organizations/Systems and Public Health Policy and Community Advocacy**
Clean water	● Ask parents and caregivers about water sources, especially if a child presents with waterborne illnesses. ● Remind parents and caregivers to conduct routine testing of well water. ● Provide anticipatory guidance on water safety after floods and during droughts, especially for families that rely on private wells.	● Monitor changes in commercial initiatives and policies with the potential to undermine water quality (eg, changes in water source, rezoning, changes in dumping policies, new business ventures, the addition of oil pipelines), and join communities to advocate for safe water with local, regional, and state government entities. ● Work with groups to expand access to clean water on Native American reservations and elsewhere.

Toxic waste sites, landfills, and incinerators	● Encourage patients and families to join with others in the community who are concerned about toxic waste sites, landfills, and incinerators. These may include
	  • Local, grassroots organizations
	  • Traditional environmental organizations (eg, League of Conservation Voters)
	  • Faith organizations
		● Encourage adolescents, parents, and caregivers to join community groups working to improve waste management.
		● Provide your expertise to communities and groups working to improve waste management.

(continued on next page)

Table 19–1 (*continued*)		
Topic	**Patient- and Family-Directed**	**Clinical Practice/Organizations/Systems and Public Health Policy and Community Advocacy**
Toxic waste sites, landfills, and incinerators (*continued*)	● Provide information about toxic waste sites in your community as well as freshwater bodies that may be heavily polluted. Refer to the Environmental Protection Agency EnviroAtlas for information on your community (https://enviroatlas.epa.gov/enviroatlas/interactivemap).	
Transportation	● Help caregivers, parents, and patients identify communities burdened by low-quality transportation, and help them work with community groups and policy makers to offer solutions such as bicycles, walking, carpooling, electric vehicle assistance, and transportation assistance. ● Provide resources at your clinic for accessing public transportation, bike shares, and other forms of active transportation.	● Get involved with policy on transportation infrastructure, and advocate for better transportation for limited-income, minoritized communities.

Table 19–1 (*continued*)		
Topic	**Patient- and Family-Directed**	**Clinical Practice/Organizations/Systems and Public Health Policy and Community Advocacy**

Quality housing as part of the built environment	● Encourage patients and families to join with others in the community who are concerned about the same health hazard. These may include
	  • Local, grassroots organizations
	  • Housing organizations
	  • Legal clinics
	  • Faith organizations
		● Identify children and adolescents who are living in unstable housing or unhealthy housing.
		● Work with local community groups to ensure that housing-remediation programs protect residents' health and meet climate goals (ie, lead remediation, adequate insulation, mold remediation, and replacement of methane gas appliances).

Exposure to lead	● Encourage parents and caregivers to have home water tested through the local water utility company. ● Recommend that parents and caregivers contact the local health departments for assistance with testing for lead paint and dust, especially after a renovation of an older home, to ensure that risk mitigation is complete.	● Conduct more frequent screenings of patients at risk for lead exposure.[20]

References

1. US Environmental Protection Agency. Learn about environmental justice. Updated September 6, 2022. Accessed February 13, 2023. https://www.epa.gov/environmentaljustice/learn-about-environmental-justice

2. Ragavan MI, Marcil LE, Philipsborn R, Garg A. Parents' perspectives about discussing climate change during well-child visits. *J Clim Change Health*. 2021;4:100048 doi: 10.1016/j.joclim.2021.100048

3. Etzel RA, ed. *Pediatric Environmental Health*. 4th ed. American Academy of Pediatrics; 2019

4. Ahdoot S, Pacheco SE, Paulson JA, et al; American Academy of Pediatrics Council on Environmental Health. Global climate change and children's health. *Pediatrics*. 2015;136(5):e1468–e1484 PMID: 26504134 doi: 10.1542/peds.2015-3233

5. Perera F, Nadeau K. Climate change, fossil-fuel pollution, and children's health. *N Engl J Med*. 2022;386(24):2303–2314 PMID: 35704482 doi: 10.1056/NEJMra2117706

6. Gauderman WJ, Urman R, Avol E, et al. Association of improved air quality with lung development in children. *N Engl J Med*. 2015;372(10):905–913 PMID: 25738666 doi: 10.1056/NEJMoa1414123

7. Cook Q, Argenio K, Lovinsky-Desir S. The impact of environmental injustice and social determinants of health on the role of air pollution in asthma and allergic disease in the United States. *J Allergy Clin Immunol*. 2021;148(5):1089–1101.e5 PMID: 34743831 doi: 10.1016/j.jaci.2021.09.018

8. Aithal SS, Gill S, Satia I, Tyagi SK, Bolton CE, Kurmi OP. The effects of household air pollution (HAP) on lung function in children: a systematic review. *Int J Environ Res Public Health*. 2021;18(22):11973 PMID: 34831729 doi: 10.3390/ijerph182211973

9. Villanueva CM, Kogevinas M, Cordier S, et al. Assessing exposure and health consequences of chemicals in drinking water: current state of knowledge and research needs. *Environ Health Perspect*. 2014;122(3):213–221 PMID: 24380896 doi: 10.1289/ehp.1206229

10. Tanana H, Combs J, Hoss A. Water is life: law, systemic racism, and water security in Indian Country. *Health Secur*. 2021;19(S1):S78–S82 PMID: 33944613 doi: 10.1089/hs.2021.0034

11. Rabin R. The lead industry and lead water pipes "a modest campaign". *Am J Public Health*. 2008;98(9):1584–1592 PMID: 18633098 doi: 10.2105/AJPH.2007.113555

12. Mascarenhas M, Grattet R, Mege K. Toxic waste and race in twenty-first century America: neighborhood poverty and racial composition in the siting of hazardous waste facilities. *Environ Soc*. 2021;12(1):108–126 doi: 10.3167/ares.2021.120107

13. American Public Transportation Association. Public transportation facts. Accessed March 13, 2023. https://www.apta.com/news-publications/public-transportation-facts

14. Pratt GC, Vadali ML, Kvale DL, Ellickson KM. Traffic, air pollution, minority and socio-economic status: addressing inequities in exposure and risk. *Int J Environ Res Public Health*. 2015;12(5):5355–5372 PMID: 25996888 doi: 10.3390/ijerph120505355

15. Hoffman JS, Shandas V, Pendleton N. The effects of historical housing policies on resident exposure to intra-urban heat: a study of 108 US urban areas. *Climate (Basel)*. 2020;8(1):12 doi: 10.3390/cli8010012

16. Swaringen BF, Gawlik E, Kamenov GD, et al. Children's exposure to environmental lead: a review of potential sources, blood levels, and methods used to reduce exposure. *Environ Res*. 2022;204(pt B):112025 doi: 10.1016/j.envres.2021.112025

17. National Center for Medical-Legal Partnership. Accessed February 13, 2023. https://medical-legalpartnership.org

18. American Board of Pediatrics. Self-assessment activities. Accessed February 13, 2023. https://www.abp.org/content/self-assessment-activities

19. AirNow. Air Quality Flag Program. Accessed February 13, 2023. https://www.airnow.gov/air-quality-flag-program

20. Pediatric Environmental Health Specialty Units. Management of childhood lead exposure. Updated September 2021. Accessed February 13, 2023. https://www.pehsu.net/Lead_Exposure.html

Part 3. Optimizing Anti-racism in Practice

Section 1. Clinical Practice

CHAPTER 20

Using Racial Equity Policy Tools to Further Anti-racism in Pediatrics

Nia Heard-Garris, MD, MBA, MSc, and Nevin J. Heard, PhD

Introduction

Typically, when individuals and organizations engage in work to dismantle racism, they emphasize personal responsibility and individual change.[1] People are often tasked with addressing interpersonal racist behaviors and the intrapsychic biases and prejudices that exist within their own mind (eg, racial stereotypes and prejudices), yet addressing the racist policies of the institutional environment is given little attention. Eliminating these racist policies could have a broader effect on the individuals working within and affected by these institutions. These outcomes include reducing the racial thoughts, attitudes, and *actions* of individuals. Specifically, individuals can engage in a more active process of identifying and eliminating racism by changing systems, organizational structures, policies, practices, and attitudes through the examination of policies with an anti-racist lens, so power is redistributed and shared equitably throughout society. Ultimately, anti-racism promotes racial equity and moves us closer to a more just society, which includes ameliorated health inequities. In this chapter, we posit that the most efficient and effective way of increasing racial equity is through eradicating racist policies and adopting anti-racist policies and we introduce a tool that can be used for this purpose.

A Review of Racial Equity Tools

Racial equity tools are at the center of anti-racist practice. These can be broadly defined as tools that prioritize racial equity in decisions about structures, policies, practices, programming, and resources.[2] Policy makers do not usually consider racial equity during policy development and implementation and thus, along with the policies themselves, perpetuate racial inequity (eg, unfair lending practices and housing segregation) and continue to serve dominant cultures. Racial equity tools should[2,3]

- Recognize sociocultural power dynamics.
- Institutionalize racial equity.
- Engage racially and ethnically diverse community members.
- Eliminate racial inequities.
- Advance racial equity.
- Mitigate unintended consequences.
- Develop mechanisms for successful and sustainable implementation and evaluation.

Racial equity tools are usually multilayered, collaborative, and promote institutional change through policy change.[2,3] This chapter focuses on the Government Alliance on Race & Equity (GARE) Racial Equity Tool because it is more generalizable to community-based organizations and various health care settings.[2]

The GARE Racial Equity Tool (Table 20–1) provides a framework for addressing anti-racism in organizational structures.[2] Although the GARE Racial Equity Tool, as a whole, is valuable, Step 4, in particular, allows an organization to identify who "benefits from or is burdened by" a decision. By asking that question, organizations can recognize and disrupt the status quo of racial inequity.

Applying an Anti-racist Policy Tool

The case study example that follows illustrates how a pediatric organization may apply the GARE Racial Equity Tool to promote anti-racism.

Table 20–1. Government Alliance on Race & Equity Racial Equity Tool	
Steps	**Set of Questions**
Proposal	What is the policy, program, practice or budget decision under consideration? What are the desired results and outcomes?
Data	What's the data? What does the data tell us?
Community engagement	How have communities been engaged? Are there opportunities to expand engagement?
Analysis and strategies	Who will benefit from or be burdened by your proposal? What are your strategies for advancing racial equity or mitigating unintended consequences?
Implementation	What is your plan for implementation?
Accountability and communication	How will you ensure accountability, communicate, and evaluate results?

Reproduced from Nelson J, Brooks L. *Racial Equity Toolkit: An Opportunity to Operationalize Equity.* Government Alliance on Race & Equity; 2016. Accessed February 13, 2023. https://racialequityalliance.org/wp-content/uploads/2015/10/GARE-Racial_Equity_Toolkit.pdf.

Case Study Example Regarding a Scheduling Policy[a]

A busy pediatric clinic in a large metropolitan city boasts a clinical volume of 150 patients per day. Your clinic is diverse, with a 50-50 payor mix of patients who have private and public insurance and who are multilingual and Multiracial. You have just been named medical director and are committed to implementing anti-racist practices within the clinic. Your first task is to evaluate the clinic's policies. You are told by several of the clinic staff that families have expressed concern about the scheduling policy. Your clinic's family scheduling policy is as follows:

"Only 2 patients from 1 family are allowed to be cared for at the clinic each day. If a family has more than 2 children, they must be cared for on subsequent days."

When other clinic staff find out that you are reviewing this policy, many people show interest and support, whereas others report that the policy is necessary as written because it was created to reduce the number of patients who miss appointments and the burnout of clinicians. There is significant concern that changes to the policy may increase so-called no-shows, so you decide to review the policy with the GARE Racial Equity Tool.

Step 1. Proposal

The first step is to review the policy. When it comes to the policy, it seems that attitudes are mixed, according to what you have learned from other clinic staff. The next step in the GARE Racial Equity Tool, data, may provide you with more insight.

Step 2. Data

Because the staff comments are about clinician burnout and the number of no-shows per family, you decide to seek out data on these concerns. The data reveal that clinicians have reported levels of burnout consistent with other clinics' with similar patient demographics. You learn that families with 3 or more children have had 3 times as many no-shows than families with 2 or fewer children. Given this information, you decide to analyze the no-show phenomenon to determine whether there are any differences by demographics, including race. You note that 60% of families with 3 or more children are from groups that have been racially minoritized, predominantly Black and Latinx[b] groups. In your review, you note that 50% of families with 3 or more children have reported having limited access to resources such as reliable transportation and stable housing. On further review, you note that 15% of white families and 85% of Black and Latinx families with 3 or more children have reported these resource barriers (ie, access to transportation and housing). Additionally, you find that there are no significant differences in the number of no-shows for families with 2 or fewer children when accounting for race.

---

[a] For the sake of this case study, one individual (ie, the medical director) applied the GARE Racial Equity Tool to review an existing policy, but ideally, this work will be done as part of a larger team or group composed of several community members, stakeholders, and people affected by the policy.
[b] In this chapter, we use *Latinx* when referring to people of Latin American origin or descent as a whole. It is a gender-neutral and gender-inclusive alternative to *Latino*. For a brief history of this term, including a rationale, refer to the book introduction.

(continued on next page)

Case Study Example Regarding a Scheduling Policy (*continued*)

Step 3. Community Engagement

Next, you review community engagement in decisions regarding the policy. In conversations with colleagues, you learn that this policy was instituted following a managerial administrators meeting in which there were no physicians, clinic staff, or families present. You believe there are opportunities to expand engagement and find the fact that physicians, clinic staff, and families were never consulted about the policy to be problematic. You plan to implement town hall–style meetings and task forces to expand community engagement regarding this policy in a future step. You also consider ways to increase community participation by offering child care during meetings, as well as offering vouchers for rideshare services, public transportation, and/or taxis.

Step 4. Analysis and Strategies

In Step 2, the data revealed that families with 3 or more children have been burdened by this policy overall; however, it may be having a particularly negative effect on Black and Latinx families, given the data on access to resources. Families with 2 or fewer children, regardless of race, and white families with 3 or more children may have been less affected by the policy. Although unintended, this policy has created a racial disparity within your clinic caused by access. You decide to set up a structure to learn from your Black and Latinx families about barriers to attending their appointments, to elevate their voices, and to ask their thoughts about a proposed plan in which families can bring all their children to a single medical visit.

Step 5. Implementation

Given the data and family and community feedback, you believe that modifying the scheduling policy is the correct action. Thus, you decide to revise the policy so families can make an appointment for more than 2 of their children within a single day. When it comes to implementation, families will be advised of the policy modification in multiple ways (eg, during the scheduling process; via email, electronic health record notifications [eg, MyChart], traditional mail, and telephone communication) and will be informed in multiple languages. Clinic staff would indicate during the appointment scheduling process whether they reminded the family of the policy modification to ensure that it is being implemented. Data on no-show appointments and clinician burnout will continue to be collected and analyzed on an ongoing basis. Additionally, you decide to pilot a public transportation and rideshare voucher program for families with 3 or more children and more than 1 no-show.

Step 6. Accountability and Communication

You believe that the most pragmatic way to begin to ensure accountability will be via a satisfaction survey sent to families, containing specific questions about scheduling and the policy change. Additionally, families will be notified about these improvement efforts via clinic town hall–style meetings or a task force they can join to bring up concerns they might have about the scheduling policy and its implementation. Results will be evaluated through the data collected in the implementation process. To ensure that communication is equitable, results will be discussed at a clinic meeting when all staff are available to be present and will be displayed in public spaces in which visuals are also incorporated to address language and literacy concerns. Results of the data will be given to families directly, where their feedback is solicited routinely.

Summary

Structural change is required to embrace anti-racism in multiple settings. This chapter has provided the key components of racial equity tools and, through a case study example, has illustrated how racial equity tools can be applied to pediatric settings. Although using racial equity tools is necessary for institutionalizing equity, this alone may not fully address the racial inequity burdening the larger community. Thus, organizational, community, and governmental transformation are simultaneously necessary for advancing anti-racism.

Because policies are not race neutral,[1] and because racial equity and anti-racism are not generally considered in the forming of policies and structures,[3] policies tend to benefit the dominant racial group. We recommend that racial equity tools be introduced early and used consistently so all decisions can be aligned with racial equity[2] and that policies and procedures be rigorously examined through an anti-racist lens to create a systemic and thoughtful approach that identifies the potential harms and benefits to whom.

Recommendations

Clinical Practice/Organizations/Systems

- Clinical organizations should create committees that analyze and act on racist policies.
- Clinical organizations should involve their broader community to play a significant role within these committees.
- Clinical organizations should track the outcomes of their work and share their findings broadly.

References

1. Kendi IX. *How to Be an Antiracist*. Bodley Head; 2019
2. Nelson J, Brooks L. *Racial Equity Toolkit: An Opportunity to Operationalize Equity*. Government Alliance on Race & Equity; 2016. Accessed February 13, 2023. https://racialequityalliance.org/wp-content/uploads/2015/10/GARE-Racial_Equity_Toolkit.pdf
3. Webb E, Sergison M. Evaluation of cultural competence and antiracism training in child health services. *Arch Dis Child*. 2003;88(4):291–294 PMID: 12651748 doi: 10.1136/adc.88.4.291

CHAPTER 21

Culturally Congruent Strategies to Build the Pediatric Health Workforce

Harolyn M. E. Belcher, MD, MHS; Marie Plaisime, Phd, MPH; and Carmel Bogle, MD

Introduction

Building a diverse, culturally responsive, and informed pediatric health workforce is essential to promoting the health and well-being of children and adolescents through patient-centered, family-engaged care. Using evidence-informed and culturally respectful health promotion strategies that lead to effective clinical care and that support shared decision-making between caregivers, patients, and pediatric health professionals is fundamental. Ensuring an understanding of the terminology and the context of words used in this chapter is essential for applying the work necessary to build a culturally aware pediatric health workforce (Box 21–1).

Current Demographics of the Pediatric Health Workforce

More than 2 decades ago, an Institute of Medicine, now known as the National Academy of Medicine, report showed that Black, Hispanic, and American Indian/Alaska Native health professionals were underrepresented compared to their distribution in the US population.[1] Black, Hispanic, and American Indian/Alaska Native populations remain underrepresented in medicine (eg, nurse practitioners, pediatricians, and psychologists).[2] Data in Table 21–1 demonstrate that *underrepresentation* in some health disciplines is more than 3.5 times less than expected on the basis of US racial and ethnic demographic characteristics. Black and Hispanic health professionals, including pediatricians, make up less than 15% of reported health professionals (Table 21–1) yet more than 30% of the US population. A recent study confirmed these disparities and created a diversity index comparing the race and ethnicity of working US citizens with the race and ethnicity of health professionals, in which a rank of "1" indicated equal representation. The study showed that the mean diversity index was 0.54 for Black health professionals and 0.34 for Hispanic health professionals.[3] Importantly, US educational trends do not project a burgeoning of a diverse pediatric and public health workforce that reflects the projected diversity of the US population.[4]

Box 21–1.

Definitions of Key Terms Used in This Chapter[a-c]

Ableism

Prejudice or bias against an individual or population that is neurodiverse. Neurodiversity may include, but is not limited to, individuals with intellectual, physical, emotional, or sensory disabilities.

Culture

Shared values, norms, beliefs, customs, foods, parenting or caregiving practices, and knowledge that shape attitudes and practices of a group.

Sociopolitical determinants of health

The systems and sectors in which we live, learn, work, play, and pray. It is estimated that the social and physical environments are associated with 50% of an individual's health. The political determinants of health include US policies and practices that directly influence allocation of resources related to the social determinants of health.[a]

Stereotype threat

Lowered performance attributable to anxiety related to stereotypes prevalent in the society and culture (eg, women perform more poorly than men in STEM subjects).[b]

Imposter syndrome

A psychological term that refers to a pattern of behavior wherein people, even those with adequate external evidence of success, doubt their abilities and experience a persistent fear of being exposed as a fraud.[c]

[a] Dawes DE. *The Political Determinants of Health*. Johns Hopkins University Press; 2020.
[b] Steele CM, Aronson J. Stereotype threat and the intellectual test performance of African Americans. *J Pers Soc Psychol.* 1995;69(5):797–811.
[c] Mullangi S, Jagsi R. Imposter syndrome: treat the cause, not the symptom. *JAMA.* 2019;322(5):403–404.

Table 21–1. Health Workforce

Characteristics	Total US Population in 2019[a] (%)	Pediatrics in 2019[b] (%)	Physicians in 2018[c,d] (%)	Nurses in 2017[e] (%)	Dentistry in 2016[f] (%)	Physical Therapy in 2018[g] (%)	Psychology in 2016[h] (%)	Occupational Therapy in 2017[i] (%)	Speech Pathology in 2018[j] (%)
African American/Black	13.4	6.2	5.0	6.2	4.3	3.6	4.0	4.1	5.1
American Indian/Alaska Native	1.3	0.3	0.3	0.4	—	0.2	—	0.2	0.4
Asian	5.9	13.8	17.1	7.5	15.8	12.9	4.0	6.0	2.3
Hispanic	18.5	7.2	5.8	5.3	5.3	8.8	5.0	6.1	6.2
Native Hawaiian/Pacific Islander	0.2	0.1	1.0	0.5	—	—	—	0.16	—
White	60.1	54.7	56.2	80.8	73.6	76.7	84.0	75.5	82.0
Unknown	—	16.2	—	—	—	—	0.1	—	—
Not listed above	—	1.5	—	—	—	—	—	—	—
With disability	13.2	—	3.1	—	—	—	—	—	—

a US Census Bureau. QuickFacts. https://www.census.gov/quickfacts/fact/table/US/IPE120219. Accessed February 13, 2023.
b Montez K, Omoruyi EA, McNeal-Trice K, et al. Trends in race/ethnicity of pediatric residents and fellows: 2007–2019. *Pediatrics.* 2021;148(1):e2020026666.
c Association of American Medical Colleges. *U.S. Physician Workforce Data.* Association of American Medical Colleges; 2020. https://www.aamc.org. Accessed February 13, 2023.
d Nouri Z, Dill MJ, Conrad SS, Moreland CJ, Meeks LM. Estimated prevalence of US physicians with disabilities. *JAMA Netw Open.* 2021;4(3):e211254.
e Smiley RA, Lauer P, Bienemy C, et al. The 2017 National Nursing Workforce Survey. *J Nurs Regul.* 2018;9(3)(suppl):S1–S88.
f Health Policy Institute. *Racial and Ethnic Mix of the Dentist Workforce in the U.S.* American Dental Association; 2021.
g Deloitte, Datawheel, Hidalgo C. Physical therapists. Data USA. https://datausa.io/profile/soc/physical-therapists#demographics. Accessed February 13, 2023.
h American Psychological Association. *Demographics of the U.S. Psychology Workforce: Findings From the 2007–2016 American Community Survey.* American Psychological Association; 2018:2.
i Deloitte, Datawheel, Hidalgo C. Occupational therapy. Data USA. https://datausa.io/profile/cip/occupational-therapy. Accessed February 13, 2023.
j Deloitte, Datawheel, Hidalgo C. Speech-language pathology. Data USA. https://datausa.io/profile/soc/speechlanguage-pathologists. Accessed February 13, 2023.

Implicit Bias

Many reasons exist for the failure of the pediatric health workforce to reflect the racial and ethnic demographics of the United States. One of the most insidious and remediable reasons may be implicit or unconscious bias. Compared to explicit bias, implicit bias occurs at an unconscious level. *Implicit bias* refers to the tendency of the brain (the temporoparietal and prefrontal lobes) to generalize cultural stereotype data. This may lead to institutional and structural racism that produces policies and practices that unfairly disadvantage groups that have been marginalized and stereotyped (refer to Chapter 3, Implicit and Explicit Biases and the Pediatric Health Professional). Examples of institutional racism include policies that

- Use standardized tests with low predictive validity that favor white middle- and upper-income populations as primary criteria for admission to college, graduate, and medical schools

- Lead to lower research funding for research relevant to disorders and conditions that affect children and adolescents from marginalized groups

- Use race-based interpretation of laboratory data such as glomerular filtration rates[5-7]

Based on decades of evidence-based cognitive behavior studies, tools to reduce implicit bias are available and should be mandated to identify and correct institutional racism in pediatric health workforce selection, training, and promotion.[8] Antibias strategies to promote a diverse pediatric health workforce may include universal, evidence-based antibias training for search and selection committee members, including diverse pediatric committee members early in the process of determining scoring and prioritizing selection criteria, which is essential.

Structural and Institutional Racism in Medical Education

How Racism Leads to Health Disparities

Racism operates in several economic, political, and cultural domains, leading to health disparities. The 2003 Institute of Medicine report *Unequal Treatment* identified vital factors to address racial health disparities experienced by Black people living in the United States.[9] Various forms of bias (ie, health professional mistrust, health professional bias, and discomfort) were found to contribute to health disparities experienced by people of color. Since that seminal report, studies have focused on the role of implicit bias in clinical settings.[10]

Research demonstrates that Black patients are less likely to receive an accurate diagnosis, quality cardiovascular care, kidney transplants, and pain medication. For example, Black men are less likely to receive invasive cardiac procedures than white patients, even when presenting with identical signs and symptoms of myocardial infarction.[11]

In pediatrics, pediatric health professionals encounter similar patterns. For example, Asian, Black, and Hispanic children are less likely to receive opioids for optimal pain reduction than their white peers.[12] The role of professional bias in the clinical decision-making process is posited as a potential contributor to disparities in treatment.

Interracial Anxiety Among Medical Students

A considerable body of literature demonstrates that exposure to different racial and ethnic groups leads to greater familiarity and positive experiences. Plant and Devine[13] posit that interracial anxiety results from a lack of positive interracial interactions with members of unfamiliar cultures and racial or ethnic groups. Public health and sociological scholars note that the lack of diversity and interracial interaction in medicine contributes to the racial disparities that disproportionately adversely affect communities of color. For example, Whitla and colleagues[14] assessed medical students from predominantly white institutions and found that students minimally interacted with other racial and ethnic groups before attending medical school. They also found that students receive inadequate instruction related to patient diversity, which negatively influences their contact with non-concordant racial and ethnic patients. Race-conscious medical education approaches in pediatrics are needed to address negative associations and the occurrence of bias between racial and ethnic populations and diseases and treatments associated with specific racial groups.

Culturally Congruent Mentoring

Culturally congruent mentoring (ie, inclusive and culturally responsive mentoring strategies for diverse scholars/mentees) provides a supportive learning environment for early-career professionals.[15] The competitiveness, pace, and uncertainty inherent in medical education often lead to feelings of *imposter syndrome* (ie, despite achieving and learning at high levels of performance, the individual feels inadequate and undeserving to be in the medical school, residency, or practice). *Stereotype threat* occurs when a learner does not achieve at expected levels because of anxiety rooted in societal and cultural expectations. Mentoring may reduce feelings of imposter syndrome and stereotype threat and may assist the scholar in negotiating their institution's culture. Effective culturally congruent mentoring builds trust and mutual respect between the mentor and the scholar. Trust in a mentoring relationship emanates from active listening, openness, and time to develop nonjudgmental understanding. These trust-building skills are vital when working across racial, ethnic, and cultural groups in which implicit biases may exist.

Enhancing Mentoring

Enhancing Mentoring is a workshop designed to strengthen culturally congruent mentoring skills of graduate and early-career professional mentors. Enhancing Mentoring focuses on 5 key areas (Figure 21–1): promoting equity, diversity, and inclusion; ensuring mutual understanding and expectations; developing academic and research goals; supporting independence, self-efficacy, and leadership; and facilitating professional development and self-advocacy.[15,16] Effective communication ensures mutual understanding and expectations through the development of SMART (**S**trategic, **M**easurable, **A**ction-oriented, **R**ealistic/relevant, and **T**ime-bound) academic, professional, and research goals. Achieving mutually agreed-on SMART goals supports the scholar's independence, self-efficacy, and professional development. Effective reciprocal communication between the mentor and scholar also ensures scholar self-advocacy.

Mentors have many roles: content expert, advocate, sponsor, coach, counselor, teacher, and professional guide. The case study example that follows exemplifies how mentoring roles may change over time. An initial content expert and teacher mentor may become a sponsor, counselor, and professional guide. Ultimately, the goal of mentoring is for pediatric health professionals to thrive and succeed.

Figure 21–1. Enhancing Mentoring Wheel

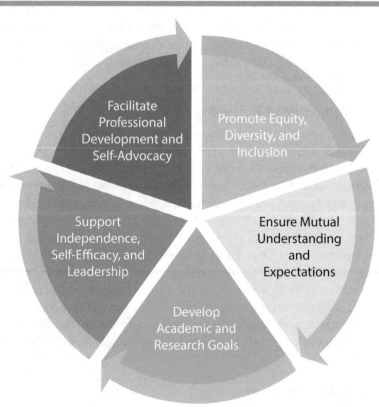

© 2019 Belcher, Stone, Wyatt
Reproduced from Wyatt GE, Belcher HME. Establishing the foundation: culturally congruent mentoring for research scholars and faculty from underrepresented populations. *Am J Orthopsychiatry*. 2019;89(3):314.

Case Study Example Using the Culturally Congruent Mentoring Model

During a medical student's second year, her father was diagnosed with terminal cancer and she requested a leave of absence to assist her family. The medical school was willing to grant her request if she could identify and participate in a research project that would compensate for the time away. The student reached out to a trusted mentor from a past research fellowship. The mentor took time to meet with the former student and understand her needs and the academic requirements for the leave of absence. The mentor worked with the student to identify an appropriate project, and together they developed SMART goals. They established periodic check-ins to ensure support and record progress on the project: writing a chapter for a neuroscience textbook. As the project progressed, the student found that she became an expert on the chapter topic. Thus, the experience gave the student relevant research and academic knowledge while allowing her the time to be with her father during his final days. The mentorship was valuable not only for the knowledge the student gained but also for the relationship the mentor promoted with the student and family. The family was touched that the mentor took time to go beyond the academic task at hand and recognized the student as someone with the potential for a successful future.

The mentor and student shared an important milestone when the student graduated medical school on time, and the mentor attended the white coat ceremony. This experience of mentorship that extended beyond the writing project enabled the student to go on to a competitive residency program, complete pediatric residency, and complete 2 subspecialty fellowships. She is now a faculty member at a prestigious medical school in the same city as her mentor. Years later, the mentor was thrilled to be invited by the former student to be a coinvestigator on the first grant proposal she wrote. It included mentoring medical students to work with adolescents who experienced disparate health outcomes following surgery. It was not lost on the mentor that the former student, now an attending pediatrician, was mentoring her mentor along with other medical students. The mentoring circle was complete.

Summary

Policies that address implicit bias across the selection, training, and promotion process in pediatrics may support the recruitment and retention of a diverse, skilled health workforce. In addition, culturally congruent and responsive mentoring strategies that build trust and open communication support the development of pediatric health professionals who acknowledge and use culturally relevant and evidence-based practices to address health disparities and promote the health and well-being of children, adolescents, and families.

Recommendations

Patient- and Family-Directed

- Build a diverse, culturally and linguistically competent pediatric health workforce to support improved patient care and communication.

Clinical Practice/Organizations/Systems

- On an ongoing basis, review policies to identify and dismantle biased recruitment, hiring, and selection criteria.

- Build a diverse, culturally and linguistically competent pediatric health workforce through continual and intentional effort.

- Use equity-based strategies to support successful hiring and retention of diverse, talented pediatric health professionals.

- Identify and employ culturally congruent mentors to enhance retention and growth of a diverse pediatric health workforce.

- Develop a mentoring team to promote academic, clinical, and career success.

Public Health Policy and Community Advocacy

- Consider mandatory antibias training to strengthen practices that promote clinician-patient trust, communication, and therapeutic relationships.

References

1. Smedley BD, Stith AY, Colburn L, Evans CH; Institute of Medicine. *The Right Thing to Do, The Smart Thing to Do: Enhancing Diversity in the Health Profession.* National Academies Press; 2001

2. National Center for Health Workforce Analysis. *Sex, Race, and Ethnic Diversity of U.S. Health Occupations (2011–2015).* Health Resources and Services Administration, US Dept of Health and Human Services; 2017:1–11. Accessed February 13, 2023. https://bhw.hrsa.gov/sites/default/files/bureau-health-workforce/data-research/diversity-us-health-occupations.pdf

3. Salsberg E, Richwine C, Westergaard S, et al. Estimation and comparison of current and future racial/ethnic representation in the US health care workforce. *JAMA Netw Open.* 2021;4(3):e213789 PMID: 33787910 doi: 10.1001/jamanetworkopen.2021.3789

4. National Center for Science and Engineering Statistics. *Women, Minorities, and Persons With Disabilities in Science and Engineering.* National Science Foundation; 2019. NSF publication 19–304. Accessed February 13, 2023. https://ncses.nsf.gov/pubs/nsf19304/digest/introduction

5. Cerdeña JP, Plaisime MV, Tsai J. From race-based to race-conscious medicine: how anti-racist uprisings call us to act. *Lancet.* 2020;396(10257):1125–1128 PMID: 33038972 doi: 10.1016/S0140-6736(20)32076-6

6. Lucey CR, Saguil A. The consequences of structural racism on MCAT scores and medical school admissions: the past is prologue. *Acad Med.* 2020;95(3):351–356 PMID: 31425184 doi: 10.1097/ACM.0000000000002939

7. Power-Hays A, McGann PT. When actions speak louder than words—racism and sickle cell disease. *N Engl J Med.* 2020;383(20):1902–1903 PMID: 32871062 doi: 10.1056/NEJMp2022125

8. Devine PG, Forscher PS, Austin AJ, Cox WT. Long-term reduction in implicit race bias: a prejudice habit-breaking intervention. *J Exp Soc Psychol.* 2012;48(6):1267–1278 PMID: 23524616 doi: 10.1016/j.jesp.2012.06.003

9. Geiger HJ. Racial and ethnic disparities in diagnosis and treatment: a review of the evidence and a consideration of causes. In: Smedley BD, Stith AY, Nelson AR, eds. *Unequal Treatment: Confronting Racial and Ethnic Disparities in Health Care.* Institute of Medicine; 2003:417–454

10. Greenwood BN, Hardeman RR, Huang L, Sojourner A. Physician-patient racial concordance and disparities in birthing mortality for newborns. *Proc Natl Acad Sci USA.* 2020;117(35):21194–21200 PMID: 32817561 doi: 10.1073/pnas.1913405117

11. Condon JV, Miller KM, Le AH, Quasem M, Looney SW. Acute myocardial infarction and race, sex, and insurance types: unequal processes of care. *Health Care Manag (Frederick)*. 2008;27(3):212–222 PMID: 18695400 doi: 10.1097/01.HCM.0000285057.32235.5e

12. Banks J, Hill C, Chi DL. Plan type and opioid prescriptions for children in Medicaid. *Med Care*. 2021;59(5):386–392 PMID: 33528236 doi: 10.1097/MLR.0000000000001504

13. Plant EA, Devine PG. The antecedents and implications of interracial anxiety. *Pers Soc Psychol Bull*. 2003;29(6):790–801 PMID: 15189634 doi: 10.1177/0146167203029006011

14. Whitla DK, Orfield G, Silen W, Teperow C, Howard C, Reede J. Educational benefits of diversity in medical school: a survey of students. *Acad Med*. 2003;78(5):460–466 PMID: 12742780 doi: 10.1097/00001888-200305000-00007

15. Wyatt GE, Belcher HME. Establishing the foundation: culturally congruent mentoring for research scholars and faculty from underrepresented populations. *Am J Orthopsychiatry*. 2019;89(3):313–316 PMID: 31070415 doi: 10.1037/ort0000417

16. Wyatt GE, Chin D, Milburn N, et al. Mentoring the mentors of students from diverse backgrounds for research. *Am J Orthopsychiatry*. 2019;89(3):321–328 PMID: 31070417 doi: 10.1037/ort0000414

Book Sharing and Children's Literature as a Strategy for Facilitating Conversations on Race

Dipesh Navsaria, MD, MPH, MSLIS

Introduction

Book sharing can play an essential role in anti-racism work with families. Fundamentally, reading books together serves several critical functions, not all of which are the exclusive domain of conversations around racism and discrimination. Sharing books offers a route for building vital elements of relational health. It is a foundation for discussions within families in which parents or caregivers can play that all-important, sense-making role for their children as they explore and wonder about the world around them. Book sharing can create a scaffold for conversations or ease the route into discussing topics, particularly if they are not necessarily easy to take on.

Although book sharing includes families reading aloud together with younger children, it can also include families facilitating book choices for older children and discussing what they are reading, even if it is not being actively read aloud by a parent or caregiver. This approach is particularly effective with adolescents and can extend to young adults.

Children, Race, Parenting, and the Role of Books

One of the initial challenges for pediatric health professionals in thinking about the role of books in their work with children on anti-racism has less to do with books and reading and more to do with what the adults around the children believe they know. The concept of *childhood innocence* has a stronghold among adults. The first step is to help adults understand that the act of talking about race will not make children suddenly begin to "see race." This adult-engendered concern is often brought up early in conversations about anti-racism work with children and needs to be handled well before moving into other conversations.

Connected to this is the notion of *color-blind parenting,* or the mistaken idea that the correct approach is to simply not bring up race. The reality is that numerous studies show that children do notice racial differences at surprisingly young ages, as young as infancy.[1,2] Moreover, when we do not offer children explanations for or ways of looking at the world, they fill the gaps by making up their own reasons that make sense on a superficial, developmentally appropriate but not very sophisticated level.

An example of this is *essentialist thinking,* or thinking that observed differences in skin color must also designate some more profound biological differences, such as in intelligence or stamina. So, for example, if a child observes that people experiencing homelessness are more likely to be people of color, they may make a false but straightforward assumption that the person is in such a situation because of some inherent reason connected to their darker skin. The more complicated but accurate elements of current and historical racism, bias, and discrimination would not occur to a younger child without some element of adult guidance. One of the core jobs of parenting and caregiving is helping children with the process of sense making, so avoiding discussions around uncomfortable topics such as race is a disservice.

Books can facilitate these conversations by offering scaffolding for discussions and offering perspectives into other worlds. Best known for this concept is Rudine Sims Bishop, who has spoken of books as serving several metaphorical roles: as mirrors, reflecting the experiences of the reader (or listener); as windows, allowing the reader to peer into the worlds of others; and as sliding glass doors, not only allowing that view but also affording the possibility to enter those worlds.[3] Some have added maps to the original concept, reflecting the idea that books can also "serve as a guide to worlds as yet unseen."[4]

The Role of the Pediatric Health Professional in Facilitating Conversations

The well-known Reach Out and Read program trains pediatric health professionals to effectively incorporate early-literacy conversations into the regular health supervision visits in the first 5 years after birth.[5] More than a book giveaway, the program focuses on supportive inquiry, coaching, reinforcement, and modeling. These interactive, family-focused frameworks offer a remarkable opportunity to not only ask about race-based conversations but also offer materials that build on these interactions.

Although a full exploration of the intervention is not possible in this chapter, a key component of it is the use of a neutral, supportive question as an opener (eg, "How often do you have a chance to read together with your child?"). This not only sets the stage by offering a subject for discussion but also signals that we are ready to listen to one of any number of responses, rather than a socially desirable but perhaps inaccurate response. This type of signaling can serve as the basis for initial trust building, which can then allow for more candid conversations around race, racism, and more.

Even if a family is not yet interested in a discussion, the indication that these topics are valid points of discussion for a health supervision visit opens the door for the possibility of future conversations. It may be that the family does not consider the topic to be relevant, that they have not yet developed sufficient trust to be able to discuss it meaningfully, or that it is not something they have even contemplated.

Of note, in keeping with other chapters of this book, discussions of race, racism, and discrimination should be universal but tailored to the needs of individual families. By no means should the assumption be made that only white families need this guidance because these discussions benefit all children and families and all children and families benefit from diverse representation in books.

The American Academy of Pediatrics policy statement "Literacy Promotion: An Essential Component of Primary Care Pediatric Practice" also makes relevant recommendations, notably the provision of "…developmentally, culturally, and linguistically appropriate books…."[6] Although early childhood is a focus of many pediatric literacy efforts, reading is critical across the full spectrum of the life span. Books written for school-aged and adolescent populations can and should also play the role of templates for discussion of these topics.

Creating Demand

Recognize that by seeking out high-quality, diverse books and advising parents to do the same, you are creating a market for such books to be written, illustrated, published, and republished. In a Reach Out and Read podcast interview with Ashley Lukashevsky, illustrator of *Antiracist Baby*, she made exactly this argument, noting how critical market demand is for publishers to take on any book project.[7]

The act of recommending these items not only lifts up the themes and ideas within them but also supports those imagining, creating, and distributing them. Make your decisions wisely.

Thoughtful Strategies for Selecting Diverse Books

There is also critical advice on avoiding well-intentioned but, ultimately, marginalizing book selections, which can reinforce cultural stereotypes, define nondominant cultures as "the other," and inadvertently exclude individuals who have been racially and ethnically minoritized from being recognized as equally likely participants in activities. Although many of these topics can be valid, important, and worthy of attention, when presented without context or as part of a limited repertoire of subjects, they can create false and reductive impressions (eg, a book depicting contemporary Native American people as routinely wearing ceremonial regalia may create or reinforce the notion that people of Native nation heritage can always be identified solely by this clothing, thereby contributing to their being "invisible" in contemporary society). Box 22–1 includes some strategies for selecting diverse books, while Box 22–2 outlines some ways for avoiding stereotypes when choosing books.

A good resource on how to counsel parents on having conversations with their children is the American Psychological Association RES (Racial Ethnic Socialization) project.[8] It not only offers a number of possible questions that parents may consider asking their child about a book they have read (eg, "Do you notice similarities or differences between the characters [and yourself]?" for younger children, "Does the book remind you of something that you've experienced in real life? Why?" for older children) but also prepares parents for questions their children may ask them (eg, a younger child may ask "Why is that person's hair different?" and an older child may ask "Why do the police shoot and sometimes kill unarmed Black people? [ie, racial profiling, police shootings]").

Box 22–1.

Strategies for Caregivers to Select Diverse and Inclusive Books

Select books that

- Include characters who share your child's race and ethnicity and your family's cultural and religious beliefs, as well as characters who do not
- Have people of color as main characters
- Provide a voice to those who rarely have one
- Tell stories that challenge myths or stereotypes (eg, *Hair Love*, written by Matthew A. Cherry and illustrated by Vashti Harrison, is about a Black father doing his daughter's hair)
- Tell stories that normalize daily life among all racial identities (eg, *Corduroy*, written and illustrated by Don Freeman, is about a Black mother and child going shopping)
- Help children and adolescents develop social action skills (eg, helping older adults, having environmental awareness, or volunteering at a soup kitchen)
- Help children and adolescents recognize inequities in social structures (eg, consider books about gender and sports within the United States or differential treatment of holidays)
- Are written or illustrated by people that have been racially and ethnically minoritized
- Are age appropriate (eg, picture books for children 5 and younger; chapter books for elementary school–aged children; chapter books for older children; longer books, novels, and graphic novels for adolescents)
- Present characters facing real-life experiences
- Showcase experiences relevant to their own (eg, *The Snowy Day*, by Ezra Jack Keats, is about a Black boy enjoying walking through his neighborhood in the snow)

Adapted from Dougé J, Jindal M. Using books to talk with kids about race and racism. HealthyChildren.org. Updated January 14, 2022. Accessed February 14, 2023. https://www.healthychildren.org/English/healthy-living/emotional-wellness/Building-Resilience/Pages/using-books-to-talk-with-kids-about-race-and-racism.aspx.

Box 22–2.

Strategies for Caregivers to Avoid Stereotypes in Book Selection

Avoid the following 5 Fs, which can overgeneralize individuals or groups of people:

- Food (eg, "Mexican" or "Chinese" cuisine)
- Fashion (eg, Native American regalia)
- Folklore (eg, tales found in numerous traditions)
- Festivals (eg, holidays such as Kwanzaa or Cinco de Mayo)
- Famous people (eg, US Civil Rights leaders in the 1960s)

Although these categories of books can be useful, they often make up the majority of books that are considered diverse. They may be used but should not be the only selections offered.

Adapted from Dougé J, Jindal M. Using books to talk with kids about race and racism. HealthyChildren.org. Updated January 14, 2022. Accessed February 14, 2023. https://www.healthychildren.org/English/healthy-living/emotional-wellness/Building-Resilience/Pages/using-books-to-talk-with-kids-about-race-and-racism.aspx.

Summary

Although there are many ways to discuss and explore race and society with children and adolescents, the route of book sharing, whether through direct reading aloud, book recommendations, or discussion, can provide a helpful framework for families to navigate these conversations. Existing early-literacy promotion programs designed for use in busy primary care practices can be a way for pediatric health professionals to incorporate guidance without adding to the burden of effectively structured yet time-limited visits. A significant pitfall to be aware of is to unwittingly reach for well-intentioned but potentially harmful content that reinforces stereotypes or marginalization, in both the books selected and the advice given to families on what to look for.

Recommendations

Patient- and Family-Directed

- Include in conversations with patients and families that books can facilitate discussion on race with children and adolescents by offering scaffolding for discussions and offering perspectives into other worlds. One approach is to use a neutral, supportive question as an opener (eg, "How often do you have a chance to read together with your child?"). This creates the opportunity for candid conversations, if families are open and willing, about topics such as race, racism, and racial identity.

- Build resources containing and referencing quality and diverse books that enable children and adolescents to see themselves and others.
- Extend the conversation about books to include children from birth to young adulthood.

Clinical Practice/Organizations/Systems

- Incorporate Reach Out and Read into your practice.
- Incorporate discussions about diverse books with all families and create places for brief documentation within health record templates.
- Work toward adoption of literacy promotion as a standard of care within your clinic or health system, with appropriate funding, support, and quality improvement.

Public Health Policy and Community Advocacy

- Work across institutions and at regional, state, and federal levels to adopt literacy promotion as a standard of care and, in particular, give care and attention toward quality and diverse books.
- Advocate for appropriate funding for literacy promotion programs in medical settings.

References

1. Kelly DJ, Quinn PC, Slater AM, et al. Three-month-olds, but not newborns, prefer own-race faces. *Dev Sci.* 2005;8(6):F31–F36 PMID: 16246233 doi: 10.1111/j.1467-7687.2005.0434a.x
2. Katz PA. Racists or tolerant multiculturalists? how do they begin? *Am Psychol.* 2003;58(11):897–909 PMID: 14609382 doi: 10.1037/0003-066X.58.11.897b
3. Bishop RS. Mirrors, windows, and sliding glass doors. *Perspect.* 1990;6(3). Article republished at: Reading is Fundamental. January 3, 2015. https://www.rif.org. Article archived at: Science Regional Library. August 2017. Accessed February 14, 2023. https://scenicregional.org/wp-content/uploads/2017/08/Mirrors-Windows-and-Sliding-Glass-Doors.pdf
4. Myers C. The apartheid of children's literature. *New York Times.* March 15, 2014. Accessed February 14, 2023. https://www.nytimes.com/2014/03/16/opinion/sunday/the-apartheid-of-childrens-literature.html?_r=0
5. Reach Out and Read. Accessed February 14, 2023. https://reachoutandread.org/about
6. High PC, Klass P, Donoghue E, et al; American Academy of Pediatrics Council on Early Childhood. Literacy promotion: an essential component of primary care pediatric practice. *Pediatrics.* 2014;134(2):404–409 PMID: 24962987 doi: 10.1542/peds.2014-1384
7. Interview with Ashley Lukashevsky, illustrator of *Antiracist Baby.* Reach Out and Read. July 30, 2020. Accessed February 14, 2023. https://reachoutandread.org/rorpodcast-season-one
8. American Psychological Association. Reading and RES: Parent Tip Tool; Choosing and Using Books to Discuss Race and Ethnicity. American Psychological Association. Accessed February 14, 2023. https://www.apa.org/res/parent-resources/reading?tab=3

CHAPTER 23

Talking With White Children and Adolescents About Racism

Margaret A. Hagerman, PhD, and Megan R. Underhill, PhD

Most importantly, white parents can play an important role in challenging the perpetuation of racism and racial inequality in the United States only if they are willing to give up some of their own white racial power by rejecting the idea that their own child is more innocent and special and deserving than other people's children are.

Margaret A. Hagerman, PhD, White Kids: Growing Up With Privilege in a Racially Divided America, *2018*

Introduction

White children and adolescents form ideas about race that are based on their everyday experiences, their interactions with others, and their observations of patterns in their social environments. Although white children certainly have ideas about race and racism, many white parents and caregivers refrain from speaking with their children about race altogether.[1-3]

Researchers have identified several reasons why white parents and caregivers avoid these conversations. First, many white parents and caregivers assume that their children do not "see race" and believe that talking about race will "upset" or bias their children.[4] Some white parents and caregivers associate race exclusively with people of color and do not recognize that white people are also a racial group. Other parents and caregivers worry about saying the wrong thing and being perceived as racist. Finally, many white parents and caregivers lack a comprehensive understanding of American history and assume that schools will address issues of race and racism with their children, freeing them from the responsibility.[3,5] However, given the current assault on racial discussions in schools, this is a fraught conclusion.

Some white parents and caregivers do speak with their children about race and racism by using color-blind messaging and promoting the idea that "we are all the same." Although unintended, color-blind rhetoric minimizes racism in the United States and naturalizes white superiority by decoupling white Americans' social, political, and economic advantages from the discriminatory policies and practices—native land seizure, the institution of slavery, and Jim Crow segregation, among others—that enabled white advantage. Color-blind rhetoric also ignores that the United States is organized hierarchically by race and that American children are racial actors within the racial order.

Although less common, recent scholarship indicates that a small contingent of "socially progressive" white parents and caregivers communicate *color-conscious* racial messages to their children. These parents and caregivers acknowledge racial inequality and frame racism as a *systemic* and *structural* problem rather than a consequence of individual-level bias. Color-conscious parents and caregivers speak with their children about their white identity, their white privilege, and the importance of white allyship.[6,7] Unfortunately, many white children do not have these discussions with their families, with some white children even growing up in families that reinforce explicit forms of white nationalism and racism.

This chapter provides insights from current social science research about how white children learn about race and discusses best practices for communicating with white children about race in ways that promote color-conscious thought and action.

Addressing Racism in Early Childhood

In contrast to conventional wisdom, white children "see" race. By the age of 3 years, they demonstrate a positive racial bias toward members of their racial group and use racial categories to reason about behavior.[8,9] Parents, caregivers, and pediatric health professionals can counter the development of racism in early childhood by increasing white children's skills at identifying and talking openly about racism. One strategy is to read children's books that feature discussions of racism, racial inequality, and anti-racist action.[10,11] Another strategy includes highlighting how racism works in daily life by pointing out racist patterns in children's and adolescents' media, everyday interactions, and dynamics in one's community.[7] Asking children questions and embracing children's curiosity about racial matters, including listening to what they have to say, are additional ways to counter the development of racist thinking and acting in white children.

Observations and Interactions in Middle Childhood

By the age of 8 years, white children learn that it is socially unacceptable to express explicit, public forms of racism. Although child-initiated racial discussions become less common during middle childhood, implicit forms of racism increase as white children's exposure to the outside world grows.[12] During this time, children notice patterns about where people from different racial groups live, work, or go to school. They talk with friends about race and bring home observations from school about racial patterns in school discipline and the racial composition of classes labeled "gifted," "advanced," and "remedial."[13–15] As they approach early adolescence, they often consume various forms of media and communicate with others in online spaces such as social media.

Because the world is larger than the family, children encounter ideas about race irrespective of whether their parents or caregivers broach the subject.[16] White parents and caregivers need to help their children contextualize and denaturalize their racial observations via discussions of the racist policies and practices that created segregated and unequal environments for Americans of color to work, live, and learn in. This type of parental and caregiver support is especially important because race-conscious education has always been underdeveloped in the US curriculum but is now under assault by conservative politicians and activists. They argue that racial discussions result in "reverse discrimination" toward white people. Given this reality, there is no better time for white children to learn, perhaps even alongside their white parents or caregivers, about the legacy of racism in the United States, how racism is perpetuated in contemporary society, and what individuals and larger social movements are doing to combat these disparities. Doing so enhances white children's social sensitivity to racial inequality and provides them with the tools to begin developing an anti-racist framework.

Power of Actions and Modeling Behavior Throughout Childhood

Modeling anti-racist action is equally as important as talking with children about racism. One crucial lesson that white parents and caregivers can impart to their children is to "care for children of color," be mindful that children of color will face racial discrimination, and speak "out and up" when aware of racist treatment.[17] Parents and caregivers can also model allyship by supporting national and local racial justice initiatives, particularly those led by people of color. They can donate their time, money, and expertise to racial justice initiatives and invite their children to join them in their work (eg, crafting signs, distributing flyers, and helping with the setup and breakdown of local events).[6,7]

Prioritizing concern for the collective good rather than acting in one's own personal, best interest is yet another strategy that parents and caregivers can use to work toward equity and challenge subtler forms of racism. When white parents and caregivers say they want to raise white children who are not racist but then use their whiteness to secure unfair advantages for their children, they reinforce the very forms of inequality they otherwise say they reject.[15] Alternatively, research indicates that some Black mothers strategize ways to boost the self-esteem and outcomes for their children while also leveraging their capital to serve and advance outcomes for their entire community.[18] The latter approach places value on community over individuals and can be harnessed to build social movements that promote social change.

Racial silence sends children and adolescents the wrong message about race; race does matter, and racism and racial inequality remain organizing forces of life in the United States, as evidenced by differential outcomes in income and wealth, education, and illness and death. White silence promotes "collective forgetting" among white people regarding issues of race and racism, hindering racial justice initiatives.[19] But white people *are* implicated in racial matters and have reaped unfair advantages because of their dominant racial position. How white people make sense of this privilege in childhood and adolescence has meaningful consequences because studies show that people's racial ideas are often difficult to change by late adolescence.[20] Indeed, racism hurts everyone, including white people. For example, research shows that white resentment toward the advancement of people of color in society can lead white people to behave in ways that undermine their best interests, such as voting against better schools, better health care, or safer gun laws.[21]

Summary

Overall, it is imperative to recognize that white children and adolescents are not too innocent, naive, or fragile to critically engage in race-related topics. As social science research with white children and adolescents clearly demonstrates, even if parents, caregivers, or other adults do not talk openly with their children about racism, childhood racial learning processes are already well underway because they grow up in a racialized society.

Recommendations

Patient- and Family-Directed

- Encourage families to become educated about America's racial history.
- Empower children to ask questions about race.
- Provide children with the tools to identify racism and misinformation about racism in their daily lives.
- Listen to children's ideas, support their racial learning, and encourage them to act as racial allies.
- Urge families to consider how choices made about how to set up a child's social environment, whether it be the schools they attend or the books they read, or the neighborhood they live in, inform their children's racial learning. Empower families to make different choices that help them align stated values with behaviors.
- Prioritize concern for the collective good.
- Encourage parents and caregivers to model anti-racist behaviors.

Clinical Practice/Organizations/Systems

- Train pediatric health professionals to apply the strategies discussed in this chapter with parents and caregivers.
- Ensure that organizations do their part to counter popular myths about white children and racism, such as the notion that white children are harmed by learning about racism.

● Support the inclusion of a curriculum in schools that critically explores racism of the past and present.

Public Health Policy and Community Advocacy

● Advocate for structural changes to laws, policies, and practices that advance racial equity.

References

1. Abaied JL, Perry SP. Socialization of racial ideology by white parents. *Cultur Divers Ethnic Minor Psychol.* 2021;27(3):431–440 PMID: 33914582 doi: 10.1037/cdp0000454

2. Hagerman MA. White families and race: colour-blind and colour-conscious approaches to white racial socialization. *Ethn Racial Stud.* 2014;37(14):2598–2614 doi: 10.1080/01419870.2013.848289

3. Underhill MR. Parenting during Ferguson: making sense of white parents' silence. *Ethn Racial Stud.* 2018;41(11):1934–1951 doi: 10.1080/01419870.2017.1375132

4. Underhill MR. "Diversity is important to me": white parents and exposure-to-diversity parenting practices. *Sociol Race Ethn (Thousand Oaks).* 2019;5(4):486–499 doi: 10.1177/2332649218790992

5. Hamm JV. Barriers and bridges to positive cross-ethnic relations: African American and white parent socialization beliefs and practices. *Youth Soc.* 2001;33(1):62–98 doi: 10.1177/0044118X01033001003

6. Heberle AE, Hoch N, Wagner AC, Frost RL, Manley MH. "She is such a sponge and I want to get it right": tensions, failures, and hope in white parents' aspirations to enact anti-racist parenting with their young white children. *Res Hum Dev.* 2021;18(1–2):75–104 doi: 10.1080/15427609.2021.1926869

7. Underhill MR, Simms L. Parents of the white awokening. *Contexts.* 2022;21(1):20–25 doi: 10.1177/15365042221083006

8. Hirschfeld LA. Children's developing conceptions of race. In: Quintana SM, McKown C, eds. *Handbook of Race, Racism, and the Developing Child.* John Wiley & Sons; 2008:37–54

9. Van Ausdale D, Feagin JR. *The First R: How Children Learn Race and Racism.* Rowman & Littlefield Publishers; 2001

10. Hughes-Hassell S, Barkley HA, Koehler E. Promoting equity in children's literacy instruction: using a critical race theory framework to examine transitional books. *Sch Libr Media Res.* 2009;12. Accessed February 14, 2023. https://eric.ed.gov/?id=EJ877497

11. Winkler EN. Why does Latino/a youth literature matter? how children and young adults learn about race. In: Henderson L, ed. *The Américas Award: Honoring Latino/a Children's and Young Adult Literature of the Américas.* Lexington Books; 2015:7–26

12. Raabe T, Beelmann A. Development of ethnic, racial, and national prejudice in childhood and adolescence: a multinational meta-analysis of age differences. *Child Dev.* 2011;82(6):1715–1737 PMID: 22023224 doi: 10.1111/j.1467-8624.2011.01668.x

13. Lewis AE. *Race in the Schoolyard: Negotiating the Color Line in Classrooms and Communities.* Rutgers University Press; 2003

14. Tyson K, ed. *Integration Interrupted: Tracking, Black Students, and Acting White After Brown.* Oxford University Press; 2011 doi: 10.1093/acprof:oso/9780199736447.001.0001

15. Hagerman MA. *White Kids: Growing Up With Privilege in a Racially Divided America.* NYU Press; 2018

16. Winkler EN. *Learning Race, Learning Place: Shaping Racial Identities and Ideas in African American Childhoods.* Rutgers University Press; 2012

17. Austin N, Underhill M, Hagerman M, Landrieu M. The power of motherhood. *E Pluribus Unum.* June 9, 2021. Accessed February 14, 2023. https://www.unumfund.org/power-of-motherhood

18. Dow DM. *Mothering While Black: Boundaries and Burdens of Middle-class Parenthood.* University of California Press; 2019

19. Mueller JC. Producing colorblindness: everyday mechanisms of white ignorance. *Soc Probl.* 2017;64(2):219–238 doi: 10.1093/socpro/spx012

20. Hagerman MA. Racial ideology and white youth: from middle childhood to adolescence. *Sociol Race Ethn (Thousand Oaks).* 2020;6(3):319–332 doi: 10.1177/2332649219853309

21. Metzl JA. *Dying of Whiteness: How the Politics of Resentment Is Killing America's Heartland.* Basic Books; 2019. Accessed February 14, 2023. https://www.basicbooks.com/titles/jonathan-m-metzl/dying-of-whiteness/9781541644960

CHAPTER 24

Racial Trauma and Trauma-Informed Practice

Camille Broussard, MD, MPH, and Nia Imani Bodrick, MD, MPH

But all our phrasing—race relations, racial chasm, racial justice, racial profiling, white privilege, even white supremacy—serves to obscure that racism is a visceral experience, that it dislodges brains, blocks airways, rips muscle, extracts organs, cracks bones, breaks teeth. You must never look away from this. You must always remember that the sociology, the history, the economics, the graphs, the charts, the regressions all land, with great violence, upon the body.

Ta-Nehisi Coates, Between the World and Me, *2015 (p10)*

Realizing the Trauma of Racism

The Concept of Racial Trauma

Since the seminal study in 1998, linking adverse childhood experiences (ACEs) and life-long health,[1] ACEs have come to include racism.[2,3] Racism is not only an adversity that affects health[4,5] but also a form of trauma that can affect other ACEs. Racial trauma or race-based traumatic stress includes overt, covert, violent, threatening, interpersonal, community-level, onetime, periodic, and/or daily experiences.[6] Further, as children and adolescents are nested within families and communities, racial trauma is often intergenerational. Caregiver experiences of racial trauma may challenge their capacity to provide an environment that buffers toxic stress.[7] Thus, trauma-informed practice is critical for pediatric health professionals to address the effects of racism while promoting resilience and well-being for these children and adolescents and families. This chapter identifies examples of historical and contemporary racial trauma in the United States to ground our understanding of the need to provide culturally and racially responsive care, illustrates how to recognize trauma symptoms associated with race-based stress, and concludes with recommendations for practice.

Historical Racial Trauma in the United States

European colonists used the concept of race as a social construct to fuel policies and laws designed to categorically displace and deprive communities of color of their rights and power. It began with the stripped sovereignty of Native American populations in

the 17th century and continued with the forced removal of millions of African populations into the transatlantic trade of people who had been enslaved. In 1830, the Indian
Removal Act authorized the forcible removal of Native American populations from their
ancestral lands to territory west of the Mississippi River; this forced displacement led to
the death of thousands of Native American people and the creation of the reservation
system for Indigenous peoples. Additionally, starting in the 1860s, Native American
children were removed from their families and confined in boarding schools designed
to erase Native American identity and promote assimilation to European-American
standards of culture. After the institution of slavery was abolished, subsequent restrictive black codes (1865–1866) and Jim Crow laws (1877–1964) were enacted to legalize
and brutally enforce racial segregation. Asian Americans have also been subjected to
traumatic incarceration with the incarceration of Japanese Americans during World
War II. Beginning in the 1990s, several states implemented immigration policies that
criminalized undocumented immigrants and prevented their use of health services,
which disproportionately affect communities from Mexico and Central America.[8] The
legacy of these historical traumas continues to affect communities today.

Contemporary Racial Trauma in the United States

Pervasive racial traumas, which have roots in the aforementioned historical traumas,
continue to occur in the United States. For example, police killings and over-policing
of Black, Indigenous, and People of Color (BIPOC) can be linked to brutal patrolling
of enslaved people and enforcement of black codes and Jim Crow laws against Black
people. This over-policing extends to disproportionality in school discipline, justice/
legal involvement, and incarceration of BIPOC adolescents.[9] Children and adolescents
have continued to be traumatized by separation from their families of origin. Recent
examples include disproportionality of Black and Indigenous children and adolescents
involved in the child welfare system and of migrant children being separated from their
families at the US-Mexico border. Additionally, secondary traumatic exposure is pervasive with increased video and image accessibility from social media, and news coverage
of killings of BIPOC individuals that is reminiscent of lynching photography[10,11] and with
increasing violence against Asian people in the context of the COVID-19 pandemic.[12]
Recognizing these historical and contemporary racial traumas is critical to understanding the context of trauma symptoms.

Recognizing Trauma Symptoms of Race-Based Stress

Trauma symptoms vary across individual children and adolescents who have experienced trauma. The FRAYED mnemonic (Table 24-1) has been adapted to describe
unique race-based traumatic stress symptoms that pediatric health professionals can
recognize when patients present for care. It is important to assess for these symptoms
as a part of trauma-informed practice and to recognize how these symptoms affect
health care interactions. Pediatric health professionals can then sensitively address and
respond to difficulties in patient interactions.

Responding to Racial Trauma

Trauma-informed practice involves *realizing* the pervasiveness and origins of trauma, *recognizing* trauma symptoms, *responding* by integrating knowledge about history and trauma into policies and practices, and *resisting re-traumatization*.[13,14] It is critical to

Table 24–1. Health Care Implications for Race-Based Traumatic Stress Symptoms		
Trauma Symptoms (The FRAYED Mnemonic)	**Race-Based Traumatic Stress Symptoms**	**Implications for Health Care Interactions**
F Frets and fear, including anxiety and chronic fear	● Fear that trauma and loss will continue for oneself and one's future generations ● Internalized feelings of fear engendered by elders' stories	● Anxiety in health care settings/offices ● Anxiety with undressing, sensitive examinations, or touch ● Anxiety with security procedures/personnel ● Avoidance of medical care and/or procedures ● Underreporting of concerns
R Regulation difficulty, including lack of self-regulation and emotional/behavioral dysregulation	● Self-destructive behavior ● Self-hatred resulting from assaults on one's sense of self ● Hypersensitivity to threat, even minimal threat ● Increased vigilance and suspicion ● Rage ● Violent behavior	● Outbursts during medical visits ● Decreased adherence to the treatment plan ● Increased medical trauma in pediatric settings/offices during examinations and/or procedures
A Attachment challenges	● Negative cognitive frames about relationships with people outside one's racial group ● General mistrust	● Delay in care seeking ● Difficulty trusting medical professionals ● Decreased buy-in for the treatment plan
Y Yelling and yawning (from overtiredness or lack of sleep); yucky feeling	● More pervasive irritability ● Oppositional behavior ● Sleep problems ● Somatic concerns	● False appearance of ambivalence toward improving one's health ● Decreased adherence ● High use of emergency department or sick visits ● "Difficult patient" label

(continued on next page)

Table 24–1 (*continued*)		
Trauma Symptoms (The FRAYED Mnemonic)	**Race-Based Traumatic Stress Symptoms**	**Implications for Health Care Interactions**
E Educational and developmental delays, with impaired learning and thinking	• Erosion of personal and cultural identities	• Difficulty engaging in motivational interviewing techniques • Difficulty identifying one's strengths
D Defeated, dissociating, or depressed feeling	• Sense of a foreshortened future • General loss of meaning and of sense of hope • Despair • Perception of the world as a hostile place • Internalized devaluation and voicelessness • Poor or altered sense of oneself	• Delay in care seeking • Difficulty asking questions of medical professionals • Underreporting of concerns • Difficulty engaging in shared-decision making • Lack of trust in the patient-professional relationship

Adapted from Common traumatic stress reactions in response to racial trauma. In: Forkey HC, Griffin JL, Szilagyi M. *Childhood Trauma and Resilience: A Practical Guide*. American Academy of Pediatrics; 2021:145.

incorporate knowledge of the aforementioned examples of racial trauma and trauma symptoms when partnering with children and families of color in practice because many will require trauma-informed care, given the pervasiveness of racial trauma. This will also require engaging and partnering with families and communities during the development of policies, processes, and a safe, built physical environment.

Patient- and Family-Directed Trauma-Informed Practice

Relational Health

To address racial trauma in pediatrics, a culture shift must occur from the traditional problem-based medical practice ("I must fix you") to a life course and relational health perspective that accounts for social determinants of health ("I must understand you so I can support you").[15] Fundamentally, this changes questioning from "What is wrong with you?" to "What has happened to you?" and "What is strong with you?" while assessing capacity for the development of a safe, stable, and nurturing caregiver-child relationship.[12,15] Practicing compassionate listening, asking open-ended questions, being mindful of body language, and using conversational interviewing skills with children and families can help pediatric health professionals build trust and foster therapeutic communication. One cannot expect to break down decades of mistrust in one medical visit; however, by demonstrating empathy during each visit, we can begin to build trust with groups that have been racially and ethnically traumatized. Acknowledgment and validation of a child's and family's experiences of racial trauma are also key in providing responsive care.[16] Further, pediatric health professionals can support families in having "the talk," which is a racial socialization message that many Black parents and caregivers have with their children about how to safely conduct themselves during interactions with police and other authority figures.[17] Caregivers may have heard the talk themselves as children and they have likely experienced their own racial trauma. We must not blame caregivers for challenges in providing safe, stable, and nurturing environments in these instances. Instead, we must invest in the caregiver-child relationship and promote positive parenting skills.[12,15] Thus, an intergenerational approach to care and healing is needed in trauma-informed practice in pediatrics.[13]

Resiliency and Racial Socialization

A trauma-informed practice should promote resiliency and well-being by identifying and building on strengths while fostering racial pride and identity. Promoting positive racial identity in children and adolescents can buffer against race-based traumatic stress and internalized racism.[18,19] Identity development is also a key developmental task of adolescence. Pediatric health professionals need to partner with families in this task. Asking about a caregiver's own sense of racial pride can initiate the conversation, followed by a developmentally appropriate conversation with the child about how they view themselves in the world and how the world views them.[16] It is important to allow children, adolescents, and families space to authentically tell their truth without invalidation. By genuinely desiring to develop relationships with these children, adolescents, and families, pediatric health professionals can promote resiliency in the face of racial trauma.

Systems-Directed Trauma-Informed Practice

Physical and Emotional Safety

One of the core elements of a trauma-informed practice is physical and emotional safety. Unfortunately, medical institutions have not historically represented safe spaces for communities of color and the vestiges of these practices have contributed to mistrust and caution when seeking health care. From an individual perspective, the act of entering a medical establishment can be stressful or triggering. Thus, an honest assessment and acknowledgment of an institution's own racial trauma history, followed by an assessment of the built physical environment, is needed before committing to becoming a trauma-informed and anti-racist institution. For example, in creating patient-centered safe spaces, an assessment of security policies is warranted. A spectrum of measures such as metal detectors, security officers/police officers, and security checkpoints may be implemented with the best of intentions. Yet limiting the use of armed security guards, reviewing restraint policies, streamlining security processes, and using clear language for explaining policies and procedures are useful techniques to reduce unintended harm.[20]

Workforce Development

Creating a culturally responsive and diverse workforce is essential for breaking down mistrust, increasing access to care, and, ultimately, reducing health disparities. A culturally responsive health care system acknowledges and incorporates the importance of culture, assesses cross-cultural relations and dynamics that result from cultural differences, expands cultural knowledge, and adapts services to meet the culturally unique needs of the population served.[21] Specific strategies include

- Hiring a diverse workforce (administrative, clinical, and ancillary staff, including security personnel) that reflects and comes from the community
- Developing organizational goals that prioritize the improvement of health services for communities that have been marginalized
- Creating and strengthening equitable and authentic partnerships with community-based organizations and agencies
- Providing culturally congruent resources

Public Health Approaches and Community Advocacy

Collaboration and Community Resilience

The Pair of ACES model[3] (Figure 24–1) of examining adverse community environments to determine needs and identify strengths can be used to develop policies and practices that build community resilience. With this understanding, many hospitals and medical practices have developed various approaches to addressing social determinants of health. These may include screening families for health-harming legal needs, colocating social services and mental health services in the medical home, medicolegal partnerships, and structural supports to connect families to needed resources.

Summary

This chapter has provided a historical and contemporary context of trauma through the lens of racial discrimination and the importance of trauma-informed care used as a universal precaution.[22] Pediatric health professionals can take action in reducing health effects from racial trauma by realizing, recognizing, and responding to racial trauma in the context of trauma-informed practice.

Recommendations

Patient- and Family-Directed

- Use the strengths-based relational health approach to trauma-informed care by assessing for and investing in safe, stable, and nurturing caregiver-child relationships to buffer the effects of racial trauma.

Figure 24-1. The Pair of ACEs Tree

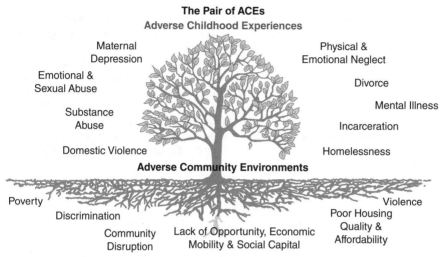

The Pair of ACEs
Adverse Childhood Experiences

Maternal Depression

Emotional & Sexual Abuse

Substance Abuse

Domestic Violence

Physical & Emotional Neglect

Divorce

Mental Illness

Incarceration

Homelessness

Adverse Community Environments

Poverty

Discrimination

Community Disruption

Lack of Opportunity, Economic Mobility & Social Capital

Violence

Poor Housing Quality & Affordability

Reproduced with permission from Ellis WR, Dietz WH, Kuan-Lung DC. Community resilience: a dynamic model for public health 3.0. *J Public Health Manag Pract*. 2022;28(suppl 1):S18–S26.

- Build safe and trusting relationships with patients and families by authentically demonstrating empathy, asking questions that try to understand patients and families, and acknowledging patient and family experiences of racial trauma.

- Promote resiliency and racial socialization by identifying and building on strengths of patients, families, and their communities.

Clinical Practice/Organizations/Systems

- Foster physical and emotional safety by first assessing and acknowledging an institution's own history with racial trauma, followed by assessing the built environment and policies that may trigger re-traumatization.

- Invest in creating a diverse, culturally and racially responsive workforce.

Public Health Policy and Community Advocacy

- Foster community resilience by empowering authentic and sustainable community collaborations and partnerships to ensure community voice remains at the center of patient care.

References

1. Felitti VJ, Anda RF, Nordenberg D, et al. Relationship of childhood abuse and household dysfunction to many of the leading causes of death in adults. The Adverse Childhood Experiences (ACE) Study. *Am J Prev Med*. 1998;14(4):245–258 PMID: 9635069 doi: 10.1016/S0749-3797(98)00017-8

2. Cronholm PF, Forke CM, Wade R, et al. Adverse childhood experiences: expanding the concept of adversity. *Am J Prev Med*. 2015;49(3):354–361 PMID: 26296440 doi: 10.1016/j.amepre.2015.02.001

3. Ellis WR, Dietz WH. A new framework for addressing adverse childhood and community experiences: the building community resilience model. *Acad Pediatr.* 2017;17(7)(suppl):S86–S93 PMID: 28865665 doi: 10.1016/j.acap.2016.12.011

4. Sanders-Phillips K, Settles-Reaves B, Walker D, Brownlow J. Social inequality and racial discrimination: risk factors for health disparities in children of color. *Pediatrics.* 2009;124(suppl 3):S176–S186 PMID: 19861468 doi: 10.1542/peds.2009-1100E

5. Trent M, Dooley DG, Dougé J, et al; American Academy of Pediatrics Section on Adolescent Health, Council on Community Pediatrics, and Committee on Adolescence. The impact of racism on child and adolescent health. *Pediatrics.* 2019;144(2):e20191765 PMID: 31358665 doi: 10.1542/peds.2019-1765

6. Carter RT. Racism and psychological and emotional injury: recognizing and assessing race-based traumatic stress. *Couns Psychol.* 2007;35(1):13–105 doi: 10.1177/0011000006292033

7. Ford KR, Hurd NM, Jagers RJ, Sellers RM. Caregiver experiences of discrimination and African American adolescents' psychological health over time. *Child Dev.* 2013;84(2):485–499 PMID: 23020184 doi: 10.1111/j.1467-8624.2012.01864.x

8. Martinez O, Wu E, Sandfort T, et al. Evaluating the impact of immigration policies on health status among undocumented immigrants: a systematic review. *J Immigr Minor Health.* 2015;17(3):947–970 PMID: 24375382 doi: 10.1007/s10903-013-9968-4

9. Welch K, Lehmann PS, Chouhy C, Chiricos T. Cumulative racial and ethnic disparities along the school-to-prison pipeline. *J Res Crime Delinq.* 2022;59(5):574–626 doi: 10.1177/00224278211070501

10. Bor J, Venkataramani AS, Williams DR, Tsai AC. Police killings and their spillover effects on the mental health of Black Americans: a population-based, quasi-experimental study. *Lancet.* 2018;392(10144):302–310 PMID: 29937193 doi: 10.1016/S0140-6736(18)31130-9

11. Downs K. When Black death goes viral, it can trigger PTSD-like trauma. PBS NewsHour. July 22, 2016. Accessed February 14, 2023. https://www.pbs.org/newshour/nation/black-pain-gone-viral-racism-graphic-videos-can-create-ptsd-like-trauma

12. Findling M, Blendon RJ, Benson J, Koh H. COVID-19 has driven racism and violence against Asian Americans: perspectives from 12 national polls. Health Affairs Forefront. April 12, 2022. Accessed February 14, 2023. https://www.healthaffairs.org/do/10.1377/forefront.20220411.655787/full

13. Duffee J, Szilagyi M, Forkey H, Kelly ET; American Academy of Pediatrics Council on Community Pediatrics; Council on Foster Care, Adoption, and Kinship Care; Council on Child Abuse and Neglect; and Committee on Psychosocial Aspects of Child and Family Health. Trauma-informed care in child health systems. *Pediatrics.* 2021;148(2):e2021052579 PMID: 34312294 doi: 10.1542/peds.2021-052579

14. SAMHSA's Trauma and Justice Strategic Initiative. *SAMHSA's Concept of Trauma and Guidance for a Trauma-Informed Approach.* Substance Abuse and Mental Health Services Administration; 2014. HHS publication (SMA) 14–4884

15. Garner A, Yogman M; American Academy of Pediatrics Committee on Psychosocial Aspects of Child and Family Health, Section on Developmental and Behavioral Pediatrics, and Council on Early Childhood. Preventing childhood toxic stress: partnering with families and communities to promote relational health. *Pediatrics.* 2021;148(2):e2021052582 PMID: 34312296 doi: 10.1542/peds.2021-052582

16. Svetaz MV, Coyne-Beasley T, Trent M, et al. The traumatic impact of racism and discrimination on young people and how to talk about it. In: Ginsburg KR, ed. Ramirez McClaine ZB, associate ed. *Reaching Teens: Strength-Based, Trauma-Sensitive, Resilience-Building Communication Strategies Rooted in Positive Youth Development.* 2nd ed. American Academy of Pediatrics; 2020:307–328

17. Anderson LA, O'Brien Caughy M, Owen MT. "The talk" and parenting while Black in America: centering race, resistance, and refuge. *J Black Psychol.* 2022;48(3–4):475–506 doi: 10.1177/00957984211034294

18. Miller DB. Racial socialization and racial identity: can they promote resiliency for African American adolescents? *Adolescence.* 1999;34(135):493–501 PMID: 10658857

19. Sellers RM, Copeland-Linder N, Martin PP, Lewis RL. Racial identity matters: the relationship between racial discrimination and psychological functioning in African American adolescents. *J Res Adolesc.* 2006;16(2):187–216 doi: 10.1111/j.1532-7795.2006.00128.x

20. Iguchi MY, Bell J, Ramchand RN, Fain T. How criminal system racial disparities may translate into health disparities. *J Health Care Poor Underserved.* 2005;16(4)(suppl B):48–56 PMID: 16327107 doi: 10.1353/hpu.2005.0081

21. Castillo RJ, Guo KL. A framework for cultural competence in health care organizations. *Health Care Manag (Frederick).* 2011;30(3):205–214 PMID: 21808172 doi: 10.1097/HCM.0b013e318225dfe6

22. Racine N, Killam T, Madigan S. Trauma-informed care as a universal precaution: beyond the adverse childhood experiences questionnaire. *JAMA Pediatr.* 2020;174(1):5–6 PMID: 31682717 doi: 10.1001/jamapediatrics.2019.3866

CHAPTER 25

Why #RepresentationMatters in Media

Nusheen Ameenuddin, MD, MPH, MPA

Introduction

Children and adolescents exist in a media-saturated world, an inevitable side effect of being born in the Information Age and growing up as digital natives, unlike earlier generations. So ubiquitous is technology that an infant's finger swipe to unlock a smartphone could well be considered a contemporary developmental milestone. Inquiring about the type, duration, and location of media use of children and adolescents during health supervision visits has been a part of American Academy of Pediatrics recommendations for pediatric health professionals since the 1990s.[1] During the COVID-19 pandemic and resultant social-distancing recommendations, educational and recreational media use increased substantially among children and adolescents as families sought alternatives to face-to-face instructional, social, and physical activities.[2]

The full effect of this enhanced media saturation on children during the pandemic has yet to be determined, but the situation has highlighted and exacerbated existing inequities in media access and representation, especially as issues related to diversity, equity, and inclusion in media can affect the mental and physical health of preadolescents.[3] For example, although we often think of media as a reflection of society, media powerfully influences its consumers as it shapes societal values; establishes norms regarding beauty, power, and behavior; and often reinforces problematic racial, ethnic, and other stereotypes, especially to impressionable young minds.

This chapter examines

- The power of media and its effects on children and adolescents, both as a reflection and an influencer of society

- The importance of representation in both entertainment and news media, on the screen and behind the scenes, especially for children and adolescents of color who have fewer examples of positive media coverage

- How to apply lessons from media literacy with an equity lens to consume, appraise, and advocate for greater diversity and inclusion in media, with suggested action items for pediatric health professionals to improve representation in media to enhance child well-being

The Power of Media

In 2010, Kaiser Family Foundation published results of a landmark survey showing that children spent more than 7.5 hours a day engaged in media use, a duration comparable to the amount of time spent at school or asleep.[4] Therefore, it is somewhat reasonable to surmise that media has an outsized influence on children and adolescents and how they view the world and themselves. With approximately 50% of children in the United States from Black, Latinx[a]/Hispanic, Asian, Indigenous/Native American, and more Multiracial backgrounds and 1 in 4 children and adolescents from an immigrant home, one might expect media to more accurately reflect this demographic shift.[5,6] Yet entertainment media primarily portrays white male characters, especially in leading and protagonist roles, who do not accurately reflect current US or world demographics, resulting in children and adolescents seeing comparatively fewer actors of color in both fictional and nonfictional roles.[7] Another study showed that, with higher media use, this disparity negatively affected the self-esteem of Black preadolescents and white girls but positively affected the self-esteem of white boys, likely because the media reinforced stereotypical roles and prioritized white male protagonists across media.[3]

The Importance of Representation in Media

Disparities in Quality and Content of BIPOC Portrayals in Media

Black, Indigenous, and People of Color (BIPOC) portrayals in media are limited and not always favorable. For example, Arab and Muslim characters are portrayed primarily in a negative light. In fact, among movies from 2017 to 2019, there were only 1.6% of speaking parts for Muslim characters.[8] Moreover, many of the characters were portrayed as terrorists or victims of oppression.[9] Actors with brown skin, often of South Asian or Middle Eastern roots, were often limited to roles such as the aforementioned. Indeed, even when Latin American creators such as Lin-Manuel Miranda worked to dispel stereotypes about his community as he wrote the musical *In the Heights*, he faced pushback from executives who wanted to play up stereotypical portrayals of Hispanic communities.[10] Disparities in award nominations and wins, made by largely white voting members, also affect actors and creators of color. April Reign created the social media hashtag #OscarsSoWhite in 2015 in response to all Academy Awards going to white nominees for the first of 2 consecutive years.[11] Even when representation is present on-screen, colorism can often play a role, in which lighter-skinned actors have been prioritized for roles over darker-skinned actors, even in ethnic majority movies such as India's Bollywood movie industry and the film version of *In the Heights*. Colorism is a practice rooted in racism and colonialism, but it is being called out more by Black, Latinx, and Asian populations in the beauty and media industries.

Increasing Diversity in Media

There have been efforts to increase diversity both behind and in front of the camera. *Sesame Street*, for example, has served as a model for diversity on-screen for decades.

---

[a] In this chapter, we use *Latinx* when referring to people of Latin American origin or descent as a whole. It is a gender-neutral and gender-inclusive alternative to *Latino*. For a brief history of this term, including a rationale, refer to the book introduction.

Musicals such as *Hamilton* have applied *color-blind casting*, which allows actors of any racial or ethnic background to play any role in a story that would otherwise feature only white characters. The 1990s saw a number of television shows created by and for Black Americans, such as *A Different World*, which was set at a fictional historically Black college and anecdotally encouraged Black children and adolescents to seek higher education.[12] More recently, shows like *Black-ish* and *Mixed-ish* have provided a platform to discuss deeper racial and societal issues in the context of upper- and middle-class Black American families in a network sitcom format. Asian American creators such as Mindy Kaling, Margaret Cho, and Eddie Huang have created television series inspired by their lives as second-generation immigrants in the United States, with Kaling acknowledging that difficulty being cast in roles led her to create her own show. Even in the superhero universe, offerings such as *Black Panther*, *Shang Chi*, and *Ms. Marvel* have provided audiences with Black and Asian superheroes, while *Rogue One* from the Star Wars franchise showed a diverse band of heroes who helped set in motion the valorous events of one of the largest, most lucrative entertainment franchises in the world. Streaming services such as Netflix and Disney Plus have created entertainment content directed at children and adolescents that feature more intentionally diverse casts that apply *color-conscious casting*, which acknowledges and amplifies the unique experiences and heritage of BIPOC actors in roles that can authentically celebrate who they are.

The examples of positive representation shared have been shown by research studies to positively influence behavior in children and favorably contribute to diversity enhancement. For example, when a group of preschool children were shown *Sesame Street* clips of BIPOC and white children playing together and then shown photos of diverse children and asked who they would want to play with in real life, the children who watched the clips of diverse groups of children playing together were more likely to choose a child of a different racial or ethnic background as a potential playmate.[13] We are also learning more about how vicarious racism and violence through media can negatively affect BIPOC children and adolescents. With the accessibility of social media and its ability to rapidly disseminate videos of real-life violent events, such as police shootings of unarmed Black adolescents, focus groups have shown that BIPOC adolescents may experience negative emotions, primarily helplessness, after exposure to this media.[14] More than 1,000 older studies that examined the effects of fictional virtual violence on children and adolescents consistently showed a connection between watching violence and experiencing increased feelings of aggression in children.[15] However, we must now also consider the detrimental effect of virtual violence on the mental and physical health of children who identify with the victims, especially when videos of Black men and boys being killed are shared widely through media.

Applying Digital Literacy and an Equity Lens to Media

Equipping children and adolescents with the ability to critically appraise media and the messages it is sending, subconsciously and otherwise, is essential to developing media literacy and applying an equity lens to its consumption. Digital and media literacy needs will continue to evolve as technology does. With this evolution, pediatric health professionals can play an important role in supporting families as they develop a media use plan and approach. Discussions can also encourage children to think more deeply about what is being presented and whether there is an overriding message, as well as whether there are perspectives not being covered or whether there is a message being conveyed that does not seem accurate or fair.

Summary

Equity, diversity, and inclusion in media is neither achieved by checking a box nor accomplished by relegating BIPOC actors to background roles. Our diverse patient populations of color deserve to have their stories and experiences front and center. As pediatric health professionals, we must advocate on every level to ensure that our next generation feels represented and included by us and the larger world, including the media that shapes so much of their lives and affects their health and well-being.

Recommendations

Patient- and Family-Directed

- Educate caregivers and patients about setting some limits on media use, encouraging caregivers to co-view media with children, and suggest prosocial media with positive portrayals of diverse characters.

- Work to diversify patient education materials to better represent and reflect the larger populations. Also, set an example by putting inclusive decorations, books, and toys into the office.

Clinical Practice/Organizations/Systems

- Advocate for improved representation in media through the following suggested 4 As action items:
  - Advocate: Speak up and take action to encourage more diverse media that reflects our younger patient populations.
  - Amplify: Share and elevate voices and perspectives of groups that have been historically excluded and, therefore, may not be well represented in mainstream media.
  - Add: Consider hiring pediatric staff who are a "cultural add" rather than a "good fit," which can perpetuate homogeneity in the workplace and does not reflect changing demographics of our patient populations, who deserve to see themselves represented not just in media but in everyday roles so they understand that "they can be what they can see."

- Assemble: Gather, display, and distribute representative materials around your workplace (eg, multicultural holiday recognition) and among staff (eg, research articles, books) to create a welcoming, inclusive, educational environment for families and staff.

References

1. Brown A; American Academy of Pediatrics Council on Communications and Media. Media use by children younger than 2 years. *Pediatrics.* 2011;128(5):1040–1045 PMID: 22007002 doi: 10.1542/peds.2011-1753
2. Jennings NA, Caplovitz AG. Parenting and tweens' media use during the COVID-19 pandemic. *Psychol Pop Media.* 2022;11(3):311–315 doi: 10.1037/ppm0000376
3. Martins N, Harrison K. Racial and gender differences in the relationship between children's television use and self-esteem: a longitudinal panel study communication research. *Communic Res.* 2012;39(3):338–357 doi: 10.1177/0093650211401376
4. Rideout VJ, Foehr UG, Roberts DF. *Generation M2: Media in the Lives of 8- to 18-Year-Olds.* Henry J. Kaiser Family Foundation; 2010
5. Population estimates show aging across race groups differs. News release. US Census Bureau; June 20, 2019. Accessed March 21, 2023. https://www.census.gov/newsroom/press-releases/2019/estimates-characteristics.html
6. Artiga S, Petry U. *Living in an Immigrant Family in America: How Fear and Toxic Stress Are Affecting Daily Life, Well-being, & Health.* Kaiser Family Foundation; 2017
7. Dunn J, Lyn S, Onyeador N, Zegeye A. Black representation in film and TV: the challenges and impact of increasing diversity. McKinsey & Company. March 11, 2021. Accessed March 21, 2023. https://www.mckinsey.com/featured-insights/diversity-and-inclusion/black-representation-in-film-and-tv-the-challenges-and-impact-of-increasing-diversity
8. Khan A, Pieper K, Smith SL, Choueiti M, Yao K, Tofan A. *Missing and Maligned: The Reality of Muslims in Popular Global Movies.* USC Annenberg Inclusion Initiative; 2021. Accessed February 14, 2023. https://assets.uscannenberg.org/docs/aii-muslim-rep-global-film-2021-06-09.pdf
9. Shaheen JG. Reel bad Arabs: how Hollywood vilifies a people. *Ann Am Acad Pol Soc Sci.* 2003;588(1):171–193 doi: 10.1177/0002716203588001011
10. In the heights: chasing Broadway dreams. *Great Performances.* PBS television. November 10, 2017
11. Ugwu R. The hashtag that changed the Oscars: an oral history. *New York Times.* February 6, 2020. Accessed March 21, 2023. https://www.nytimes.com/2020/02/06/movies/oscarssowhite-history.html
12. Luckie MS. I went to a Black college because of "A Different World." BuzzFeed News. October 26, 2015. Accessed March 21, 2023. https://www.buzzfeednews.com/article/marksluckie/i-went-to-an-hbcu-because-of-a-different-world
13. Fisch SM, Truglio RT. *"G" Is for Growing: Thirty Years of Research on Children and* Sesame Street. Lawrence Erlbaum Associates; 2001
14. Heard-Garris N, Ekwueme PO, Gilpin S, et al. Adolescents' experiences, emotions, and coping strategies associated with exposure to media-based vicarious racism. *JAMA Netw Open.* 2021;4(6):e2113522 PMID: 34129023 doi: 10.1001/jamanetworkopen.2021.13522
15. Christakis DA, Hill D, Ameenuddin N, et al; American Academy of Pediatrics Council on Communications and Media. Virtual violence. *Pediatrics.* 2016;138(2):e20161298 PMID: 27432848 doi: 10.1542/peds.2016-1298

CHAPTER 26

Positive Youth Development as an Anti-racist Strategy

Merrian J. Brooks, DO, MS; Daniela Brissett, MD; and Kenneth R. Ginsburg, MD, MS Ed

Reframing Adolescence as a Period of Opportunity

Adolescence, including preadolescence, is a time of profound opportunity when youth (aged 10–18 years) must have positive experiences that will shape them into contributing young adults. They are natural explorers who deserve adult nurturance and guidance as they examine the world and seek meaningful roles within it. Yet too many people associate adolescence with problems or risk behaviors. When it comes to youth in populations that have been racially and ethnically minoritized, subsequently referred to as *minoritized youth* for ease of reading, society is often trained to think of these youth as *high-risk*, creating a deficit-focused lens through which they are viewed. This is deeply undermining to their potential and may squander the opportunity that adolescence offers.

Celebrating Development, in Which Thriving Is the Goal

Positive youth development (PYD) provides pediatric health professionals with guiding principles to create an environment in which all youth can maximize adolescence to develop to their full potential. Rooted in the belief that youth are experts in their own lives, PYD involves caring adults who support critical features of adolescent development, including preadolescent development. We shift from adults preventing or fixing problems to adults supporting youth in building skills to foster relationships and meaningful participation in their communities.[1] Crucial to this approach is the investment in growth, which occurs as a youth acquires the skill set and confidence to ultimately explore on their own.[2] Fundamentally, PYD highlights a youth's strengths, not risks, by improving opportunities for independence, leadership, and connection.[3]

Several PYD models exist, but a specific model that is integrated with resilience-building principles describes 8 developmental factors for caring adults to nurture to help youth flourish, known as the 8 Cs (Box 26-1). Research has shown that the more we incorporate these skills into the development of youth, the better prepared they are for adulthood.[4] The theory of PYD is rooted not in being satisfied with the *absence of risk* but in setting *thriving* as the goal.

Box 26–1.

The 8 Cs of Positive Youth Development and Resilience That Pediatric Health Professionals Can Nurture

1. **Confidence:** Listen for and build on youth's (aged 10–18 years) existing strengths to build confidence. Youth gain confidence when they regard themselves as deserving and their destiny as within their control.
2. **Competence:** Communicate with youth in ways that allow them to set the agenda and reach their own conclusions. Lectures backfire. We must talk with youth, not at them, serving as facilitators to help youth make wise decisions.
3. **Character:** Acknowledge that youth are doing well and suggest that they have contributions to make to their families, schools, and community environments. Create an environment in which all are accepted as they come.
4. **Connection:** Support family bonding, school engagement, and healthy relationships with peers. By focusing on building supportive and trustworthy relationships, we thereby enhance our own connection with youth.
5. **Control:** Provide opportunities for youth to learn to solve problems they had previously and felt they could not handle. Further, support parents and caregivers to implement appropriate discipline and monitoring strategies.
6. **Coping and stress management:** Build skill sets with positive coping strategies to give youth productive, meaningful choices about how to deal with life stressors.
7. **Contribution:** Honor youth's contributions by valuing them as experts on themselves, thereby influencing the programs and services designed to meet their needs. Help them build a sense of meaning and purpose through experiencing how much they can matter to others.
8. **Critical consciousness:** Support each youth in navigating experiences with a critical eye to recognize that stereotypes do not define their identity or potential.

Based on principles from Ginsburg KR, Mackey Andrews S. The 7Cs: an interdisciplinary model that integrates positive youth development, resilience-building strategies, and trauma-sensitive practices. In: Ginsburg KR, ed. Ramirez McClain ZB, associate ed. *Reaching Teens: Strength-Based, Trauma-Sensitive, Resilience-Building Communication Strategies Rooted in Positive Youth Development.* 2nd ed. American Academy of Pediatrics; 2020:15–18.

All youth deserve to be viewed through the PYD lens, but youth of color may have the most to gain from our collective shift in focus. The PYD approach was developed in the 1980s in response to the risk model that had become central to the way that health, education, and juvenile legal systems approached adolescence. It supports youth development by

- Providing unbiased, solid support to youth while highlighting and advocating for strong connections with natural supports (ie, parents or caregivers, family, friends) in their lives

- Helping youth optimize opportunities to explore their interests and assets
- Working hard to lower barriers to belonging that are disproportionately experienced by minoritized youth

The end goal is not simply creating a racism-free environment but creating a world in which all youth can thrive and meet their potential. Creating an equitable world and eliminating the undermining forces of racism are critical steps in reaching this larger goal.

Adolescent development is an ongoing process shaped by interactions with family, peers, and the community, including pediatric health and other youth-serving professionals. What does it mean to meaningfully connect to youth regardless of their backgrounds? It is not measured in minutes or hours spent with them but made purposeful by the exploration of what we love about youth.

Confronting Personal Biases to Create Authentic Connections

Unconscious biases can get in the way of creating meaningful connections. Although biases are universal to the human condition and may exist to simplify people's lives through mental shortcuts, they can form the basis of prejudices that harm our relationships, which are at the root of PYD. Unconscious bias can, for example, lead us to subconsciously expect that minoritized youth lack the strengths that promote thriving. This expectation directly undermines our ability to authentically connect with youth and causes us to dismiss them. How can we truly connect with someone if we do not acknowledge their potential?

Every interaction with youth necessitates that pediatric health professionals reflect on our unconscious biases. One way to do this is to gather a history that elicits the youth's strengths (Table 26-1).[5] Doing so positions us to communicate in a way that recognizes and builds on these strengths. Anti-racist work highlights empathy and humanization. Focusing on youth's strengths gives us perspective to genuinely connect with youth as whole people, something youth of color are often denied. Youth deserve to experience authentic connections as often as they can.

In addition to strengthening our relationships with youth, we must remind families, caregivers, and trusted adults that they still matter. We do our best work when we promote deep familial and cultural connections. If we take the role of caring adults seriously, we must simultaneously understand our very powerful role as people who can separate families. We must understand the disproportionality within the child welfare system and do our best to check and recheck biases that may influence the escalation of an advocacy case. We must do the anti-racist work to try to overcome the forces rooted in structural racism that fracture the connection between youth and their families. Examples of such forces, among many, include policies that over-incarcerate parents and caregivers, cause premature death of grandparents, promote poverty, and encourage grueling work schedules.

Table 26–1. Strengths-Centered History Taking for Pediatric Health Professionals	
Say This...	**Not That...**
About Trust	
I may ask you questions today that you're not yet ready to answer and that's OK. I have to earn your trust.	For me to provide care, you must answer all my questions today.
What would you like me to know about you?	What happened to you?
About Achievement	
You did X; therefore, Y happened and I see your strength. *(Pause for collective reflection)*	You are amazing.
This can feel overwhelming, but remind yourself that this can't really hurt you.	If you don't perform well, it can ruin your life.
About Solution Building	
How do you think this problem could be solved?	Let me fix it.
You have not been able to *yet*.	You can't.
About a Bad Experience	
I appreciate you for sharing how that felt for you. I hear that it hurts you.	I understand.
You will get through this.	I will fix this for you.
About Stress	
To think as much as you do is a strength. You'll be able to handle this as you think through a solution.	You worry too much.
About Seeking Support	
You deserve to feel better, and your reaching out to me, and your loved ones, shows strength.	A strong person can handle this.
About Reactivity	
You have earned the right to be angry. You have a superpower to see trouble coming and react quickly to it. Your challenge is to know when to use this superpower and to better understand when it might get in your way.	You have an anger problem.
When Feeling Unheard	
I'm sorry I did that. Thank you for letting me know how that affected you.	You misunderstood because that's not what I meant.

Table 26–1 (*continued*)	
Say This...	**Not That...**
About Parents, Caregivers, and Trusted Adults	
The adults in your lives are here to listen to your views and to help guide decisions that are ultimately your own. We encourage you to share your experiences with your parents [or caregivers] and trusted adults because you are valued and deserving of support.	You're old enough that your parents [or caregivers] are no longer needed to help you make decisions.

Based on principles from Ginsburg KR. The language of resilience. In: Ginsburg KR, ed. Ramirez McClain ZB, associate ed. *Reaching Teens: Strength-Based, Trauma-Sensitive, Resilience-Building Communication Strategies Rooted in Positive Youth Development*. 2nd ed. American Academy of Pediatrics; 2020:191–196.

Providing Opportunities and Setting High Expectations

Optimizing opportunities is about giving every youth a bona fide chance to act on their own behalf. When pediatric health professionals acknowledge each youth as the expert in their own life, we implicitly recognize their strength and minimize any shame that comes from feeling as if they are being fixed. This does not mean that we are unaware of the struggles they face or that we believe they already have all the solutions; rather, it positions us as facilitators who support them as they consider how best to navigate the world. It means we regard youth as problem-solvers rather than problems to be solved, inherently holding them to high expectations. It may be that the worst outcome of a problem is not the struggle itself but the adults' low expectations of youth that follow the challenge. Positive youth development insists that "problem-free is not fully prepared" and that a youth's problems should not define them.[6] Experiencing challenges is natural; a youth's ability to overcome these challenges is what generates irreplaceable developmental lessons.

Youth thrive when they have opportunities to explore the world, master their environment, and connect with caring adults. This optimal development cannot occur without a strong sense of belonging. Youth from historically marginalized groups experience barriers to belonging that stem from low expectations and a series of lived experiences. For example, a young high-performing Latina may earn her place at a top-ranked university. But if she simultaneously receives messages that she is not very smart, she may live with the daily fear that she is an imposter, as described by Steele and Aronson.[7]

Youth feel the burden of societal stigma and stereotypes. Youth are exposed to both subtle and overt messaging about the value and expectations of different ethnic and racial groups, which shapes how they make meaning of their racial and cultural heritage. Negative messages, often manifesting as low expectations and undermining ideas, can lead to internalized racism (ie, internalized negative feelings, ideas, or stereotypes about oneself caused by regular experiences of racist microaggressions and macroaggressions).

Promoting Critical Consciousness: A Requirement for Addressing Racism

Models that promote thriving must acknowledge the weight of racism on adolescent development. To meet this imperative, Svetaz and colleagues added the theory of critical consciousness to PYD models, which is an "empowering, strengths-based, non-expert directed approach that fosters insight and active engagement in solutions to challenge inequity."[8,9] It allows youth to learn the role that social, political, and economic forces and their related systems, structures, and institutions have on developmental outcomes. Pediatric health professionals should take the time with each youth to acknowledge how racism is affecting their life and their sense of self. Building solutions starts with institutions doing the anti-racist work of understanding and combating how youth and people of color are labeled, treated (microaggressions), and systemically cast out. It also includes helping a youth sort through these experiences with a critical eye so they understand that stereotypes and generalizations do not define their identity or potential.

We can teach that internalized racism comes from unfounded and unfair prejudices that have been allowed to persist in society. Knowing this helps youth understand that these ideas are not true, so they may discard them. For non-minoritized youth, it means prompting them to critically question how stereotypes influence their understanding and expectations of others and what they can do to overcome the urge toward internalized supremacy: internalized racism's equally untrue but powerful counterpart. Increasing critical consciousness intersects with other principles of PYD in that the pursuit of social justice is a strength we should help youth master. Critical consciousness gives youth, especially minoritized youth, an opportunity to meet other positive developmental goals by enhancing connection through diversity, self-confidence despite stereotypes, and the character and competence gained through working toward social justice.

Summary

Positive youth development is an ideal approach to youth interactions that pediatric health professionals can use in our offices and programs as we commit to the practice of anti-racism and pursue the state of equity. It supports all youth to develop into thriving natural explorers, a task as meaningful as when an infant learns to move or a toddler learns to communicate. We do our part by being caring and connected adults; optimizing youth-led solutions that enhance competence, autonomy, and mastery; and decreasing barriers to belonging. We advocate by preparing others to nurture the 8 developmental outcomes that help prepare youth to thrive as adults.

Recommendations

Patient- and Family-Directed

- Cultivate an authentic partnership by actively listening to youth and by providing prompts and discussion points relating to their lived experiences.
- Address obstacles by using strengths-based rather than punitive strategies.
- When providing advice and counseling, reinforce the belief that youth know themselves best and are in control of their growth by using patient-centered models such as motivational interviewing.

Clinical Practice/Organizations/Systems

- Integrate regular, youth-friendly patient/client climate reviews. This approach might mean meeting youth in the reception area with surveys or randomly calling families after visits to ensure that patients feel safe, respected, and free from discrimination in your system.
- Provide regular continuing education, including case studies, that focus on eliminating discriminatory communication from all interactions with youth.
- Implement racially diverse, community-reflective youth advisory boards for programs and practices. This approach provides organizational accountability to youth and tangible developmental opportunities.

Public Health Policy and Community Advocacy

- Partner with grassroots youth-led and youth-serving organizations to connect youth to opportunities to build critical consciousness.
- Remove policies that punish, shame, or attempt to frighten youth as a means to promote behavior change. Instead, focus on learning and high expectations.
- Build the maintenance of youth recreation and skill development into public policy as a tool to promote strength development in all youth no matter their family incomes. This might include youth summer programs, community centers, job subsidies, art classes, and vocational programs.

References

1. Youth.gov. Interagency Working Group on Youth Programs develops common language on positive youth development. Accessed February 15, 2023. https://youth.gov/feature-article/interagency-working-group-youth-programs-develops-common-language-positive-youth
2. Lerner RM, Almerigi JB, Theokas C, Lerner JV. Positive youth development: a view of the issues. *J Early Adolesc*. 2005;25(1):10–16 doi: 10.1177/0272431604273211
3. Ginsburg KR. *Building Resilience in Children and Teens: Giving Kids Roots and Wings*. 4th ed. American Academy of Pediatrics; 2020 doi: 10.1542/9781610023863

4. Svetaz MV, Barral R, Kelley MA, et al. Inaction is not an option: using antiracism approaches to address health inequities and racism and respond to current challenges affecting youth. *J Adolesc Health*. 2020;67(3):323–325 PMID: 32829758 doi: 10.1016/j.jadohealth.2020.06.017

5. Ginsburg KR. The SSHADESS Screening: A Strength-Based Psychosocial Assessment. In: Ginsburg KR, Ramirez McClain ZB, eds. *Reaching Teens: Strength-Based, Trauma-Sensitive, Resilience-Building Communication Strategies Rooted in Positive Youth Development*. 2nd ed. American Academy of Pediatrics; 2020:225–228

6. Pittman KJ, Irby M, Tolman J, Yohalem N, Ferber T. *Preventing Problems, Promoting Development, Encouraging Engagement: Competing Priorities or Inseparable Goals?* Forum for Youth Investment; 2003

7. Steele CM, Aronson J. Stereotype threat and the intellectual test performance of African Americans. *J Pers Soc Psychol*. 1995;69(5):797–811 PMID: 7473032 doi: 10.1037/0022-3514.69.5.797

8. Svetaz M, Coyne-Beasley T, Trent M, et al. The traumatic impact of racism and discrimination on young people and how to talk about it. In: Ginsburg KR, Ramirez McClain ZB, eds. *Reaching Teens: Strength-Based, Trauma-Sensitive, Resilience-Building Communication Strategies Rooted in Positive Youth Development*. 2nd ed. American Academy of Pediatrics; 2020:307–328

9. Jemal A. Critical consciousness: a critique and critical analysis of the literature. *Urban Rev*. 2017;49(4):602–626 PMID: 29657340 doi: 10.1007/s11256-017-0411-3

The Role of Pediatric Health Professionals in Promoting Equity and Child Development

Joannie Yeh, MD

Promoting Equity and Child Development

There are different approaches to talking with children and adolescents about racism and about how factors such as access to health care, education, economic stability, and a healthy environment affect them and the people around them. These factors, referred to as *social determinants of health*, are greatly influenced by racism. Families may not always know how to begin the conversation or to help their child or adolescent understand and process their feelings when they encounter discrimination. Pediatric health professionals can provide parents and caregivers with age-appropriate and factual resources to offer advice on managing personally mediated and observed racism, tips on discussing stories in the media or incidents at school and in the community, and suggested resources for further learning.

We can prepare ourselves for these discussions by first learning and understanding how racism affects peoples' health[1] and exploring how modern medicine has been influenced by racism.[1] Understanding the direct impact of racism on the health of our patients, such as how Black children are more likely to experience poorly controlled asthma than white children[2] or how devices such as forehead thermometers are less accurate for Black children than for white children,[3] can help us better frame these conversations.

The sections that follow highlight opportunities to promote family and child or adolescent awareness of diversity and equity at every health supervision visit. Please refer to Chapter 1, Moving Toward Health Equity, for discussions about health equity and Chapter 11, Neurodevelopmental Disorders and the Impact of Racism, for discussions about children with functional needs.

Birth to 6 Months of Age

As families are joyfully cuddling their newborn baby, diversity and equity may not be at the forefront of anyone's mind or among the questions about feeding, pooping, and sleeping. During this time, the pediatric health professional can reflect on how racism affects infant and maternal mortality risks and their own internal and external biases. In addition, parents or caregivers may want advice on choosing books to add to their home library and/or ways to integrate language and culture as their baby grows and develops.

Effectively responding to these queries provides an excellent opportunity to recommend diverse cultural stories, author backgrounds, character depictions, and family activities.

Six Months to 2 Years

Starting at the age of 6 months, infants may react when they see someone with different skin tones than their caregivers'.[4] Parents and caregivers need to reassure children that encountering different skin tones or facial structures is expected. The family can also harness a child's curiosity and understanding of various cultures by cultivating a diverse environment through the integration of books, dolls, and toys containing characters with varying skin tones; a diverse doll family; and other toy characters with different skin tones. In addition, bilingual parents and caregivers can use languages to talk and sing to their child. Families can also use this opportunity to reflect on the diversity within their circle of friends and to think about ways to expand their network.

Two to 5 Years

At about 2 years of age, children start to internalize the bias they observe in the world and to adopt the same behaviors.[5] Around the same time, children in populations that have been racially minoritized begin to experience discrimination because of their skin color. Pediatric health professionals can urge parents and caregivers to expose children to various cultures. Opportunities for this exposure can come through books or children's shows that sprinkle in words from another language and showcase families from different cultures. It can also be accomplished by naming colors and counting in another language with their children. Adults can also set an example by trying foods from different cultures and modeling a positive reaction.

Real-life Vignette

Some parents/caregivers may say, "Oh, our family is very mixed; my child will be fine." Yet studies show that Multiracial families still experience biases internally within their family and externally from other sources.[6,7] This comment presents a moment for the pediatric health professional to praise the parent/caregiver for raising their child in a diverse family environment, to be aware of opportunities to explore how others might treat people differently because of their skin color, and to notice and celebrate our differences.

Five to 11 Years

By school age, children practice the biases they perceive in real life or movies and develop a strong sense of justice. Although the media can be a positive source of diversity, parents and caregivers can also use it to explore biases. For example, when all the main characters in a show have one skin tone, adults can point this bias out to children and then have a conversation about it. Parents and caregivers can continue using the strategies mentioned earlier. Pediatric health professionals can suggest that adults begin with what their child knows. Ask questions about who they are playing with at school, what books they are reading, what shows they are watching, and what other children are saying about current news events. Stress honesty in conversations with children. Talk about how sometimes things are unfair, but we can choose how we act or respond and can make the world better by being kinder toward others. Discuss how we can be mindful about talking with people who look different from us and come from different cultures.

Many studies have shown that among Black, Native American, and Hispanic adolescents, those who develop a strong ethnic identity experience decreased risk for alcohol and drug use, improved body image, better academic success, and more positive mental health outcomes.[8-13] Parents, caregivers, and patients can be encouraged to investigate their heritage, read books with characters and historical figures of their heritage, and bolster a sense of ethnic identity and pride through discussions about history, food, and language.

Giving patients a space to ask questions allows pediatric health professionals to provide factual responses. For example, a patient might ask a very common question, "Why do people say Black Lives Matter, because don't all lives matter?" We can share that the differential treatment, even in health care, has affected health outcomes for Black and Hispanic children. If this patient has asthma, we can connect with them by explaining that everyone, even doctors, must reflect on how we can treat all people fairly for optimal asthma outcomes.

Adolescence and Older

From sixth grade onward, adolescents, including preadolescents, will have formulated solid opinions and can usually express them clearly. Parents/caregivers can harness their adolescent's wisdom at this age and ask them what they know and what their peers in school are talking about. Pediatric health professionals can advise parents/caregivers to

- Be honest about the news, and ask their adolescent for their opinion about it. What do they think about other family members' strong opinions?
- Notice together that some things people or the media say are unfair.
- Reflect together on an experience to which they, as an individual or a family, wish they could go back and say or do something differently, such as not making a racist joke or not staying silent when they observed unfair treatment.

Besides continuing the strategies suggested earlier, there may be opportunities for high school and college-aged students to join culture-based clubs and to participate in advocacy efforts, which could be on social media, in the neighborhood, or through their schools.

Real-life Vignette

After being queried about experiences of racism, a mother responds that her adolescent's school is very diverse and that it "doesn't have any racism." Until this part of the conversation, her son is quiet, but he quickly jumps in: "Oh yes, there is; some of the kids say racist things all the time." As pediatric health professionals, we can encourage parents and caregivers to explore with their adolescents their observations, how these situations make them feel, and how they handle them. We can also talk about how to be an "upstander," or someone who speaks up when someone else says something racist, sexist, or inappropriate in other ways. A quick way to be an upstander is to interrupt the moment and ask a clarifying question, such as "I didn't think that was funny. How's that funny again?" or "Wait, can you explain what you meant when you said that?" This strategy provides a pause for the bully to reflect on their words while calling out the remark in a way that prevents situational escalation.

Summary

Pediatric health professionals are uniquely positioned to offer counseling on the vital role of diversity in child and adolescent development with patients' families. Having shared goals and values increases the chance to engage with families and help raise kind and fair children. We can encourage our parents and caregivers to model behavior and speech that embrace diversity. We can also guide our patients and families on strategies and discussion topics to help their children celebrate differences, notice biases, and prepare to be upstanders.

Recommendations

Patient- and Family-Directed

- Learn how racism affects the health of our patients.
- Recommend diverse book titles and character/doll toys with different skin colors.
- Explore different cultures through food, shows, toys, language, and events.
- Encourage children to celebrate differences, notice biases, and share their observations.
- Brainstorm and practice ways for children and adolescents to be upstanders.

References

1. Trent M, Dooley DG, Dougé J, et al; American Academy of Pediatrics Section on Adolescent Health, Council on Community Pediatrics, and Committee on Adolescence. The impact of racism on child and adolescent health. *Pediatrics*. 2019;144(2):e20191765 PMID: 31358665 doi: 10.1542/peds.2019-1765

2. Guilbert T, Zeiger RS, Haselkorn T, et al. Racial disparities in asthma-related health outcomes in children with severe/difficult-to-treat asthma. *J Allergy Clin Immunol Pract*. 2019;7(2):568–577 PMID: 30172020 doi: 10.1016/j.jaip.2018.07.050

3. Bhavani SV, Wiley Z, Verhoef PA, Coopersmith CM, Ofotokun I. Racial differences in detection of fever using temporal vs. oral temperature measurements in hospitalized patients. *JAMA*. 2022;328(9):885–886 PMID: 36066526 doi: 10.1001/jama.2022.12290

4. Quinn PC, Lee K, Pascalis O, Tanaka JW. Narrowing in categorical responding to other-race face classes by infants. *Dev Sci*. 2016;19(3):362–371 PMID: 25899938 doi: 10.1111/desc.12301

5. Perszyk DR, Lei RF, Bodenhausen GV, Richeson JA, Waxman SR. Bias at the intersection of race and gender: evidence from preschool-aged children. *Dev Sci*. 2019;22(3):e12788 PMID: 30675747 doi: 10.1111/desc.12788

6. Atkin AL, Jackson KF, White RMB, Tran AGTT. A qualitative examination of familial racial-ethnic socialization experiences among Multiracial American emerging adults. *J Fam Psychol*. 2022;36(2):179–190 PMID: 34516156 doi: 10.1037/fam0000918

7. Franco MG, O'Brien KM. Racial identity invalidation with Multiracial individuals: an instrument development study. *Cultur Divers Ethnic Minor Psychol*. 2018;24(1):112–125 PMID: 28650181 doi: 10.1037/cdp0000170

8. Morris SL, Hospital MM, Wagner EF, et al. SACRED Connections: a university-tribal clinical research partnership for school-based screening and brief intervention for substance use problems among Native American youth. *J Ethn Cult Divers Soc Work*. 2021;30(1):149–162, 149–162 PMID: 33732098 doi: 10.1080/15313204.2020.1770654

9. Brook JS, Pahl K. The protective role of ethnic and racial identity and aspects of an Africentric orientation against drug use among African American young adults. *J Genet Psychol*. 2005;166(3):329–345 PMID: 16173675 doi: 10.3200/GNTP.166.3.329-345

10. Lisse AA, Hochgraf AK, McHale SM. Weight concerns in Black youth: the role of body mass index, gender, and sociocultural factors. *J Res Adolesc*. 2022;32(4):1341–1353 PMID: 34751485 doi: 10.1111/jora.12692

11. Miremadi D. Strong racial identity can boost academic resilience. *Women High Educ*. 2014;22(7):22–23 doi: 10.1002/whe.10481

12. Rivas-Drake D, Seaton EK, Markstrom C, et al; Ethnic and Racial Identity in the 21st Century Study Group. Ethnic and racial identity in adolescence: implications for psychosocial, academic, and health outcomes. *Child Dev*. 2014;85(1):40–57 PMID: 24490891 doi: 10.1111/cdev.12200

13. Ledesma RJ. *Ethnic Identity Statuses and Latino/a Mental Health Outcomes*. Marquette University; 2017

CHAPTER 28

Helping Minoritized Youth Resist Racism

Janie Victoria Ward, EdD

Introduction

Systemic racism, racialized police brutality, and racial bias in neighborhoods and schools, exacerbated by a worldwide pandemic, have highlighted racial health disparities nationwide. Black children and adolescents have been especially hard-hit. Race-based stressors, including racial stereotyping, prejudice, epithets, and, more subtly, microaggressions,[1] adversely affect academic performance, motivation, and retention.[2]

Pediatric health professionals, particularly school health service professionals (ie, school nurses, pediatricians, and school counselors) play an essential role in helping students stay healthy and reach their academic potential. Because racism is a risk factor in child development,[3,4] all pediatric health professionals must understand how racial and ethnic protective factors serve to support the psychosocial development of youth (children and adolescents) from populations that have been racially and ethnically minoritized, subsequently referred to as *minoritized populations* for ease of reading, and to reduce the negative effects of racial bias and discrimination. Pediatric health professionals across racial and ethnic identities are situated along a wide continuum of attitudes that reflect different levels of race awareness. Some adults in these positions have not thought much about race. Others have little experience talking openly about the influence and consequences of racism with children of color and their families. Preparing pediatric health professionals who have a minimal appreciation of racial and ethnic identity or have little awareness of the negative effects of racism on development demands that those of us in clinical practice resist being silent toward or avoiding these issues. Knowledge acquired in academic courses and in diversity, equity, and inclusion workshops can equip pediatric health professionals with the requisite skills to better support youth in minoritized populations. Navigating the rising rates of mental health struggles associated with race-based stress calls for effective resistance responses and resistance supports to optimize resilience in childhood and adolescence.

Racial Socialization in Families

To orient children to their social environment and racial and cultural identities, parents and caregivers provide interpretive lenses through which children make sense of the world and their place in it. We live in a Eurocentric society dominated by whiteness, and although children are not born racist, most white children are "parented into racism."[5] The neighborhoods, friendship circles, places of worship, and athletic teams of white Americans are often homogenous. As a result, white parents and caregivers are less likely to discuss race and racism with their children. Race is something that belongs to other (nonwhite) people. Thus, race talk in white families is often indirect, unintentional, subtle, and inadequate.[6] White parents and caregivers minimize racism; they do not recognize it because they do not experience it, and they often discount the experiences of those who do. Because of color-evasive socialization practices, white youth often lack the ability to talk honestly about race. As a result, they fail to learn how to identify exclusionary practices, challenge the normativity of whiteness, or develop the tools to combat racial inequality. Refer to Chapter 23, Talking With White Children and Adolescents About Racism.

Parental and caregiver socialization messages directed toward youth in minoritized populations (eg, Indigenous, Asian American and Pacific Islander, and Latino youth) vary. Some parents and caregivers emphasize racial and ethnic identity, whereas others stress heritage and culture. Most of the published research to date focuses on Black families, and when it comes to racism, Black parents feel that to be forewarned is to be prepared. They recognize the importance of teaching children to resist internalizing racial stereotypes and negative social pressures.[7] Racial socialization research within Black families reveals parental messages that emphasize preparation for bias, racial affirmation and pride, and gender-specific concerns (eg, the vulnerabilities of Black boys in regard to policing practices), as well as messages about cultural history, traditions, and heritage.[8] Across a variety of families of color, positive racial and ethnic identities in children have been linked to higher resilience, self-efficacy, and self-esteem[9]; academic success[10]; and positive psychosocial and health outcomes. Racial socialization messages have been found to improve mental health.[11] In their studies of depression, Davis and Stevenson suggest that Black adolescents who receive messages about racial identity that challenge prevailing mainstream narratives of racial inferiority are better prepared to cope with bias and discrimination.[12]

Developmental Stages to Consider When Talking About Race

Messages about how race works are best delivered in developmentally and age-appropriate ways. Children as young as preschool age notice and ask questions about race. They see physical differences, and even at an early age, they learn which skin color is preferred and valued in society and which is not.[13] The early childhood years are a critical time to instill pride and to prevent the internalization of racism.[14] Racial and cultural representation in books, videos, and film act as mirrors for children and can encourage positive identity and a sense of belonging. When pediatric health professionals ignore children's questions about race at these ages, children conclude that race talk is taboo and that racial inequality does not exist or does not matter. By adolescence, youth have constructed their own beliefs about race, and with advancing cognitive skills, they can begin to think critically about the interpersonal dynamics of racism, sexism, and classism. At this age, culturally different youth want to learn about the history of their own people, they are aware of differences in dominant cultural perspectives and their own group's culture, and they can identify discrepancies between what significant adults (eg, family, teachers, religious figures) say and do about racial inequalities.[14,15]

Of central concern to adolescents are questions of personal and group identities: *Who am I?* and *Where do I belong?* Adolescents also tend to have a strong sense of fairness and justice and to look for places to voice their concerns about the injustices they learn about and witness. They develop the capacity to understand fully how cultural and institutional racism, internalized superiority, and internalized oppression shape people's lives. Working on social justice issues especially appeals to adolescents who have been marginalized and are making sense of their place in society. Such work can help adolescents align their sense of *what is* with *what should be.*

Messages transmitted about race must appreciate intersectional dimensions of social identity (eg, gender identity, sexual orientation, and social class) because these dimensions shape how we view ourselves and how others view and treat us. For example, how society treats a Black cisgender girl from an upper-income family may differ significantly from how we treat a transgender adolescent who is of Puerto Rican descent and experiencing homelessness.

Variances in racial socialization exist within groups who, while phenotypically read as Black, are culturally distinct. For example, Afro-Caribbean or African families may think differently about their racial realities than African Americans who share a heritage rooted in slavery and historical discrimination. In some families of color, race talk may be downplayed or deemed too overwhelming for children. In contrast, in other families, messages might overemphasize the effects of race and racism on life chances.[16] Black children growing up in white families,[17] Multiracial children, and displaced children have unique racial socialization challenges. Issues may arise and intersect with identity, belonging, and the child's effort to negotiate a sense of "between-ness."[18] Latino immigrant families include additional messages to children that emphasize staying safe, understanding their documentation status, showing ethnic pride, anticipating stereotypes and discrimination, and self-advocating.[9] Overall, studies suggest that darker-skinned youth are subject to bias and discrimination in qualitatively different ways than lighter-skinned children.

Resisting Racism

The 4-Step Model

Children who face multiple adversities hunger for adults who are purposeful in helping them develop the competencies to overcome the negative effect of gender bias, ethnic prejudice, and racial discrimination.

The following 4-step model (*see it, name it, oppose it, replace it*) can facilitate coping, build psychosocial strengths, and establish practical resistance responses to bias. The original model emerged from studies of child-rearing practices in African American families.[7] This model promotes psychosocial resilience by helping children identify and navigate social pressures, stay connected to their cultural knowledge and legacy, and, when necessary, challenge mainstream knowledge claims.

The first step of the model is helping children appropriately detect and interpret potentially racist situations they have observed or experienced (*see it*). This includes identifying recurring attitudinal and behavioral patterns across different contexts and imagining alternatives. In the second step (*name it*), talking clearly, competently, and confidently about race is essential. At this step, pediatric health professionals might ask "Tell me more about what happened. Why do you think they said [or did]…?" or "Is there another way to think about this?" An accessible and shared vocabulary is required so children can ask questions and speak honestly about the emotional impact of racism. Naming it acknowledges and supports children's race-related emotions (eg, fear, fury, powerlessness) as they arise, however painful they may be. As we name it, we can encourage children to speak up if it is safe enough to do so or to seek support from others if it is not. In the third step (*oppose it*), we help children develop effective skills and dispositions for pushing back against racism and standing up for the values that uplift and empower us all. Oppositional acts can occur at multiple levels: individual, collective, and institutional. Effective resistance responses include decision-making capacities and problem-solving techniques, the emotional intelligence required to handle race-based affect and resolve race-based conflicts,[19] a strong self-concept, racial self-efficacy, sociopolitical awareness, and the ability to self-advocate.[7] The final step (*replace it*) is about healing from the injuries of racism. We help children replace the debilitating effects of racism by replenishing the psychic energy needed to repeatedly adapt and resist. In some families, religious beliefs provide coping strategies that upend racist systems and beliefs. For others, exposing the youth to activities that promote a positive racial and ethnic identity, teaching them about the struggles that their cultural group has faced and overcome, or sharing family stories about individuals and communities standing up to injustice in the past are strategies that empower and replenish the spirit of resistance. Youth have a long history of participating in everyday acts of resistance to promote social change. Multiracial youth coalitions have become catalysts of resistance by banding together to protest police brutality, fighting for the rights of LBGTQ+ people of color, protesting voter suppression, and calling attention to the environmental racism destroying their communities.

How Pediatric Health Professionals Can Further Assist Youth of Color to Resist Racism Effectively

Unacknowledged implicit bias and racial stress negatively affect youth in minoritized populations. Supporting students' mental and social-emotional health in school settings calls for allies (eg, teachers, pediatricians, social workers, and other adults) to become aware of, honest about, and attentive to issues of race, power, and injustice by resisting color evasiveness and silence about racism in youth's lives. We cannot expect the youth and families who have been most traumatized by racism to navigate this alone. All of us need to improve our racial literacy, diversify our surroundings, educate ourselves about the diverse ethnic and immigration histories of the youth we serve, and help them counter racism with messages and resources they can use to create resistance strategies that are effective, empowering, and within their control.

Summary

Racism is a risk factor in youth development. Pediatric health professionals can play an important role in assisting families of color to support their youth as they confront the negative effects of racial bias and discrimination. Variances in racial socialization exist across families of color. Messages focus on racial and ethnic identity, cultural values, traditions, and, for many groups, an attention to racism. Talking about racism should occur in ways that are age and developmentally appropriate. The 4-step model can assist youth in minoritized populations as they build psychosocial strengths and coping strategies and establish practical and responsible resistance responses to racial bias.

Recommendations

Patient- and Family-Directed

- Empower children and families of color to understand, prepare for, and resist the negative effects of racial bias and discrimination.

- Transmit proactive messages about cultural identities to help youth resist internalizing racial stereotypes and engender racial and ethnic affirmation and pride.

- Support parents and caregivers by sharing age-appropriate and developmentally appropriate books, videos, and films that highlight cultural histories, explore racial inequality, and affirm racial and ethnic identities (refer to Chapter 22, Book Sharing and Children's Literature as a Strategy for Facilitating Conversations, and Chapter 25, Why #RepresentationMatters in Media).

- Empower patients and families with strategies for navigating the challenges of racism that children in minoritized populations may encounter.

References

1. Banks BM, Cicciarelli KS, Pavon J. It offends us too! an exploratory analysis of high-school based microaggressions. *Contemp Sch Psychol*. 2020;26(2):182–194 doi: 10.1007/s40688-020-00300-1

2. Levy DJ, Heissel JA, Richeson JA, Adam EK. Psychological and biological responses to race-based social stress as pathways to disparities in educational outcomes. *Am Psychol*. 2016;71(6):455–473 PMID: 27571526 doi: 10.1037/a00403220

3. Sanders-Phillips K, Settles-Reaves B, Walker D, Brownlow J. Social inequality and racial discrimination: risk factors for health disparities in children of color. *Pediatrics*. 2009;124(suppl 3):S176–S186 PMID: 19861468 doi: 10.1542/peds.2009-1100E

4. Trent M, Dooley DG, Dougé J; American Academy of Pediatrics Section on Adolescent Health, Council on Community Pediatrics, and Committee on Adolescence. The impact of racism on child and adolescent health. In: Trent M, Dooley DG, Dougé J, eds. *Adolescent Health: A Compendium of AAP Clinical Practice Guidelines and Policies.* American Academy of Pediatrics; 2020:331–344 doi: 10.1542/9781610024310-part06-ch22

5. Sullivan JN, Eberhardt JL, Roberts SO. Conversations about race in Black and white US families: before and after George Floyd's death. *Proc Natl Acad Sci USA.* 2021;118(38):e2106366118 PMID: 34518224 doi: 10.1073/pnas.2106366118

6. Rockquemore KA, Laszloffy T, Noveske J. It all starts at home: racial socialization in Multiracial families. In: Brunsma DL, ed. *Mixed Messages: Multiracial Identities in the "Color-blind" Era.* Lynne Rienner Publishers; 2006 doi: 10.1515/9781685857608-014

7. Ward JV. *The Skin We're In: Teaching Our Children to Be Emotionally Strong, Socially Smart, and Spiritually Connected.* Free Press; 2000

8. Lesane-Brown CL. A review of race socialization within Black families. *Dev Rev.* 2006;26(4):400–426 doi: 10.1016/j.dr.2006.02.001

9. Ayón C. Talking to Latino children about race, inequality, and discrimination: raising families in an anti-immigrant political environment. *J Soc Social Work Res.* 2016;7(3):449–477 doi: 10.1086/686929

10. Wang MT, Huguley JP. Parental racial socialization as a moderator of the effects of racial discrimination on educational success among African American adolescents. *Child Dev.* 2012;83(5):1716–1731 PMID: 22717004 doi: 10.1111/j.1467-8624.2012.01808.x

11. Neblett EW Jr, Hudson Banks K, Cooper SM, Smalls-Glover C. Racial identity mediates the association between ethnic-racial socialization and depressive symptoms. *Cultur Divers Ethnic Minor Psychol.* 2013;19(2):200–207 PMID: 23647330 doi: 10.1037/a0032205

12. Davis GY, Stevenson HC. Racial socialization experiences and symptoms of depression among Black youth. *J Child Fam Stud.* 2006;15(3):293–307 doi: 10.1007/s10826-006-9039-8

13. Caughy MO, O'Campo PJ, Randolph SM, Nickerson K. The influence of racial socialization practices on the cognitive and behavioral competence of African American preschoolers. *Child Dev.* 2002;73(5):1611–1625 PMID: 12361322 doi: 10.1111/1467-8624.00493

14. Swanson DP, Cunningham M, Youngblood J II, Spencer MB. Racial identity development during childhood. In: Neville HA, Tynes BM, Utsey SO, eds. *Handbook of African American Psychology.* Sage Publications; 2009:269–283. Chapter republished at: University of Pennsylvania ScholarlyCommons. Accessed February 15, 2023. https://repository.upenn.edu/gse_pubs/198

15. Derman-Sparks L, Phillips CB. *Teaching/Learning Anti-racism: A Developmental Approach.* Teachers College Press; 1997

16. Williams AD, Banerjee M. Ethnic-racial socialization among Black, Latinx, and white parents of elementary school-age children. *J Soc Issues.* 2021;77(4):1037–1062 doi: 10.1111/josi.12493

17. Smith DT, Juarez BG. Race lessons in Black and white: how white adoptive parents socialize Black adoptees in predominately white communities. *Adoption Q.* 2014;18(2):108–137 doi: 10.1080/10926755.2014.895465

18. Baden AL, Steward R. The cultural-racial identity model: a theoretical framework for studying transracial adoptees. In: Javier RA, Baden AL, Biafora FA, Camacho-Gingerich A, eds. *Handbook of Adoption: Implications for Researchers, Practitioners, and Families.* Sage Publications; 2007:90–112 doi: 10.4135/9781412976633.n7

19. Stevenson HC. *Promoting Racial Literacy in Schools: Differences That Make a Difference.* Teachers College Press; 2014

Part 3. Optimizing Anti-racism in Practice

Section 2. Organization/Systems

CHAPTER 29

Best Practices in Diversity Management

Joy A. Lewis, MSW, MPH, and Rhodora Osborn, JD, LLM

Introduction

A diverse and engaged workforce is critical to the success of any health care organization. In this chapter, we explore why people in leadership positions should invest time and resources toward creating a diverse and inclusive work culture. An inclusive environment ensures equitable (ie, fair and equal) access to resources and opportunities for all. We discuss the potential benefits of an inclusive environment and highlight the actions that can undermine it and lead to recruitment and retention challenges for your organization.

Building a Culture of Respect

Employees expect to be treated with and to reciprocate respect in the workplace.

Building a culture of respect starts at the most senior levels of leadership within any organization. Senior leaders set the tone by their actions and their modeling of behaviors that they want to be demonstrated in other leaders, including mid-level managers and directors. The ultimate goal is to cascade these behavioral expectations throughout the organization, down to the unit or practice level. Increasingly, the workforce reflects the demographic diversity in society writ large, albeit not as evident at executive levels.[1] If teams are to succeed, achieve high levels of respect, and enjoy a healthy work environment, leaders can consider the following actions:

- Clearly articulate the organization's priorities related to diversity, equity, and inclusion. According to Press Ganey workforce-engagement data from fall 2021, there is a correlation between an organization's values and actions around diversity, equity, and inclusion and its employee retention.[2]

- Commit to diversity in programming, governance, and staff, among other factors. For example, ensure a diverse slate of candidates for every open position. Research shows that diverse boards and leadership teams make better decisions, leading to better overall performance and higher profit margins.[3]

- Celebrate diversity of all kinds. Diversity falls along many dimensions, such as race and ethnicity, gender identity, sexual orientation, disability, age, and immigration status, among others. Find opportunities to bring visibility to the range of diverse individuals and talents in the workplace and thereby engender respect for each other.

- Lead with cultural humility. An openness to learn about the unique set of talents and skills, characteristics, background, and prior experiences that each person possesses is a proven strategy to foster trusting, respectful, and healthy working relationships.

● Practice active listening skills. Being present and available for each other is essential for creating a culture of respect. Leaders should model and practice leading with questions, listening from a place of openness, and not opposing from a place of ego.

It is important to inform employees that there is zero tolerance for disrespect in the workplace. Reporting protocols should be clearly and regularly communicated to employees.

Antidiscrimination and Harassment Policies

Any organization, regardless of size, should have clear policies in place that prohibit discrimination and harassment. For smaller practices, this could be a 1-paragraph statement informing everyone that discrimination and harassment will not be tolerated; therefore, any reported conduct will be dealt with accordingly. The Equal Employment Opportunity Commission has outlined general antidiscrimination and harassment policy tips for small businesses.[4] For larger organizations or health systems, this effort could be part of a broader equal employment opportunity program that includes an easy-to-understand policy on preventing and eliminating harassing conduct in the workplace. This policy should highlight its importance, define the scope of its appli-cation, define the responsibilities expected of the manager and other parties, provide examples of prohibited conduct or behaviors, and detail the reporting and investigation process.

Of note, well-written policies are only as good as their implementation. Similarly, antidiscrimination and harassment policies are only as good as the implementation of other human resources policies on topics such as nepotism and favoritism. Favoritism is a form of workplace inequality that must be addressed at the outset. If based on an employee's protected characteristics, favoritism at the workplace could be illegal. For example, if one employee notices another be assigned more desirable tasks or be excused from unproductive behaviors, they may form an assumption that the other employee is favored. Due consideration must be given to employee perceptions about favoritism or nepotism in the workplace because inattention to these concerns could undermine diversity and inclusion efforts, foster conflict among employees, harm productivity, and, ultimately, affect morale. If these concerns are left unaddressed, an organization may end up being confronted with an exodus of employees or, worse, legal issues. Organizational leaders and managers must be mindful that day-to-day decisions and policies could result in unfair treatment or exclusion of others. One way to manage this is for organizational leaders and managers to foster and maintain a professional environment that actively discourages any kind of unfair treatment.[5]

Importance of Training

Medium to large health systems conduct new-hire training sessions for staff and man-agers and additional, periodic training for newly promoted supervisors or managers. In addition, some organizations mandate training on preventing discrimination and harassment in the workplace. In this context, organizational core values and behavioral expectations are shared and education about policies on code of conduct, favoritism, nepotism, discrimination, and harassment is delivered. Managers and supervisors are also educated on their roles and responsibilities in preventing discrimination and harassment and what to do if they receive a report of such an incident in the workplace. In smaller practice areas, a hiring manager can easily have a conversation with new hires about respect as an impor-tant core value, setting expectations about how the new hires should conduct themselves and the importance of respecting differences and always treating their colleagues fairly. This set of expectations could be as simple as being polite and collegial to each other or recognizing and appreciating others regardless of their roles in the organization. In this same conversation, the hiring manager can encourage staff, depending on their comfort level, to speak directly to the person involved or to seek support to address disrespectful behaviors at work. A hiring manager must also share that discrimination and harassment are prohibited conduct; therefore, any incident experienced or observed must be reported immediately so it can be addressed promptly and appropriately.

In addition to training staff in compliance, it is equally important to train staff about implicit bias. Several sources, including the American Public Health Association, the Centers for Disease Control and Prevention, and diversity, equity, and inclusion scholars, view implicit bias as *the act of applying attitudes toward people or associating stereotypes with them without conscious knowledge of doing so.*

Implicit bias is something all people possess. It can be advantageous, protective even, when put to good use. Left unchecked, the negative impacts of this bias include toxic work conditions, limited professional growth opportunities, and poor health outcomes. In health care organizations, it is common for individuals from historically marginalized communities to experience implicit and explicit biases. Each organization needs to develop a carefully crafted plan to identify and mitigate the harmful effects of implicit and explicit biases at the interpersonal and organizational levels. Investing in mandatory inclusive-leadership training has the potential to raise awareness about bias and provide actionable strategies to guard against it in the workplace. When bias goes unaddressed, it saps the organization of its full potential (refer to Chapter 3, Implicit and Explicit Biases and the Pediatric Health Professional).

Reporting Concerns

In smaller organizations, staff should know to bring their concerns about discrimination or harassment directly to their supervisor unless the concerns are about the supervisor. Staff should be informed that in this situation, they need not follow the chain of command and can connect with their human resources representative. In large organizations in which an equal employment opportunity office or a dedicated hotline is in place, inform employees about it. This is an option for them to confidentially and anonymously report inappropriate behaviors, including harassment and discrimination. Being able to report concerns is one of the key components of an informed, mindful, and safe culture in a highly reliable organization. Employees should be assured that their reports via compliance lines are carefully reviewed and promptly addressed.

Summary

Respect is necessary in a healthy work environment. Regardless of the size of an organization, its leaders must set the right tone, listen from a place of openness, and create an environment in which mutual respect among colleagues is the expectation. Establishing discipline to maintain a diverse and inclusive culture is important for many reasons, including brand recognition, improved organizational efficiency, and workforce recruitment and retention.

Recommendations

Clinical Practice/Organizations/Systems

- As leaders, prioritize actions that promote an inclusive, diverse, and respectful work environment.
- Understand that accountability is important for behaviors that are misaligned with organizational expectations.
- Implement consistent communication and antibias training, which are necessary for maintaining an inclusive culture.
- Create safe, organizational pathways to ensure an environment in which employees, particularly those from historically marginalized communities, feel empowered to report disrespectful and discriminatory behaviors.

References

1. The Leverage Network. Inequity starts at the top. February 2021. Accessed February 15, 2023. https://theleveragenetworkinc.com/inequity-starts-at-the-top-wp-2
2. Press Ganey study uncovers impact of diversity and equity on retention. News release. Press Ganey; October 27, 2021. Accessed February 15, 2023. https://www.pressganey.com/news/press-ganey-study-uncovers-impact-of-diversity-and-equity-on-retention
3. Banham R. Momentum builds for more women on boards. Forbes. December 10, 2019. Accessed February 15, 2023. https://www.forbes.com/sites/insights-kpmg/2019/12/10/momentum-builds-for-more-women-on-boards/?sh=5556a96215b0
4. Equal Employment Opportunity Commission. Harassment policy tips. Accessed February 15, 2023. https://www.eeoc.gov/employers/small-business/harassment-policy-tips
5. Kloefkorn S. Favoritism and nepotism: managing favoritism in the workplace. eSkill Talent Assessment Platform. February 5, 2019. Accessed February 15, 2023. https://eskill.com/blog/favoritism-nepotism-workplace

CHAPTER 30

The Role of Quality and Safety in Furthering Health Equity

Julia M. Kim, MD, MPH; Meghan Drayton Jackson, DO, MBOE; and Rahul Shah, MD, MBA

For care to be considered high quality, it must be equitable. Inequitable care is low-quality care and must be treated as such.

National Academy of Medicine[1]

Introduction

Equity is 1 of 6 goals for improvement in health care quality, in addition to safety, effectiveness, timeliness, patient centeredness, and efficiency, as outlined in 2001 by the Institute of Medicine (IOM), now known as the National Academy of Medicine.[2] Although this sentinel approach to health care quality was introduced more than 20 years ago, progress has been inadequate to address the disparities in health care.[1] There is a need for health professionals to shift from thinking about equity as one area to be improved to thinking about it as being embedded across all domains and efforts in quality and safety.[3] We have yet to implement a standardized approach to address this consistently.

In 2003, the IOM report *Unequal Treatment: Confronting Racial and Ethnic Disparities in Health Care* revealed inequities in the quality of care delivered to populations that had been racially and ethnically minoritized and that had limited incomes across clinical domains and organizational levels.[4] Recommendations to reduce inequities included "[promoting] equitable care and [collecting] and [reporting] data on disparities."[4] The 2009 IOM report *Toward Health Equity and Patient-Centeredness: Integrating Health Literacy, Disparities Reduction, and Quality Improvement* highlighted the role of quality improvement (QI) in addressing health literacy and reducing inequities.[5] Also, in 2009, the IOM report *Race, Ethnicity, and Language Data: Standardization for Health Care Quality Improvement* offered recommendations to standardize data collection on race, ethnicity, and language preference to improve quality and eliminate disparities.[6] Despite these calls to action and the broad availability of resources, less than 20% of pediatric hospitals currently use these data for improvement.[7] Similarly, few clinics in the ambulatory setting currently use these data for improvement, although the National Committee for Quality Assurance has set goals to incentivize health plans toward equity with recent requests for public reporting of Healthcare Effectiveness Data and Information Set quality measures stratified by race and ethnicity.[8]

The annual Agency for Healthcare Research and Quality *National Healthcare Quality and Disparities Report* in 2021 revealed continued inequities in health care quality related to race, ethnicity, and socioeconomic status (SES).[9] Households with limited incomes received worse care than households with high incomes for more than half the quality measures.[9] Although there have been improvements in health care over time, there continue to be significant inequities in all quality domains. Black, Hispanic, American Indian, and Alaska Native populations received worse care than white populations for 36% to 43% of quality measures.[9] Asian and Native Hawaiian/Pacific Islander populations received worse care for 28% of quality measures.[9]

The American Academy of Pediatrics has identified the need for QI to address the impact of racism on pediatric and adolescent outcomes and to evaluate quality, safety, and patient experience data by race to improve disparities.[10] In 2021, the National Academy of Medicine published *An Equity Agenda for the Field of Healthcare Quality Improvement*, highlighting the need to centralize equity in discussions about quality of health care and when conducting QI at the patient and health system levels.[1] Quality and safety play a crucial role in dismantling racism and furthering health equity. In this chapter, we review the evidence and describe action steps that pediatric health professionals and teams can take to achieve health equity in the context of quality and safety.

Align Quality, Safety, and Health Equity Principles and Frameworks: Use Quality and Safety Tools to Address Health Equity

Quality and safety frameworks, principles, and tools can be used to advance health equity. In 2010, the IOM updated its conceptual framework for categorizing health care quality and measuring disparities.[3] Equity was highlighted with value as a dimension across all other quality domains and introduced new aspects of quality, including access, care coordination, and health system infrastructure capabilities. This updated framework was developed to inform quality measurement, data collection, and reporting of disparities in health care quality.

Donabedian's model is a foundational framework for evaluating and measuring quality and safety and has been successfully applied in health care and other settings.[11] This approach to measuring the quality of care is defined by structure, process, and outcomes and can be used to identify and assess inequities in quality and safety. **Structural** aspects of quality are important to identify and measure as contributing factors to inequities, including neighborhood factors, access to care, health insurance, facilities, equipment, human resources, and organizational structures impacted by systemic racism. Inequities in care **processes**, including technical and adaptive aspects of care delivery, are important to measure, such as adherence to guidelines or communication between health professionals and patients, which can be affected by implicit and explicit biases.

Quality **outcomes** such as illness, death, hospitalizations, quality of life, functional status, cost, and satisfaction should also be evaluated for disparities by race, ethnicity, and language preference.

Key patient safety principles can be applied to advance health equity. These include a systems-thinking approach, a learning system approach (ie, learning from one's mistakes and creating a safe space to openly discuss meaningful events), development of a culture of safety and emphasis of teamwork, clear communication, openness about errors, development of training and staff, and engagement of patients and families.[12,13] A systems-thinking approach can be applied to embed an equity lens to promote the identification and breakdown of systemic racism across organizations, from clinical care to data analytics and health information technology, finance, patient/family experience, environmental services, or human resources.[14] A learning system approach can promote transparency, reliability, measurement, and continual improvement and learning, with the normalization of open discussions and language for discussions about race and racism in health care.[15] Developing a culture of safety aligns with developing a culture of equity, which creates a foundation for a just culture. Multidisciplinary teams and collaborators should include experts in racism and engage patients and families. As with patient safety, training should be required to emphasize everyone's role in furthering health equity and developing a workforce with the knowledge, competencies, and tools to result in improvement.

Quality and safety frameworks and principles can be applied in evaluating and measuring health equity. Health equity should be considered at each step when applied to quality and safety efforts.

Practice Equity-Focused Quality Improvement: Ensure That Quality Improvement and Patient Safety Efforts Are Not Furthering Disparities in Care

An equity lens should be embedded in all aspects of quality and safety improvement and applied to each step in the frameworks for improvement, such as the Institute for Healthcare Improvement Model for Improvement or the Lean Sigma DMAIC (**D**efine, **M**easure, **A**nalyze, **I**mprove, **C**ontrol) framework.[16,17] Equity-Focused Quality Improvement (EF-QI) is QI that is centered around equity and focused on action to improve health disparities.[18] It integrates equity through each step of the QI project and highlights the needs of populations impacted by inequity.[18] Table 30–1 highlights the call to action for applying an equity lens to quality and safety with specific strategies for practicing EF-QI. Key strategies for EF-QI include

- Identifying disparities by stratifying existing quality measures and prioritizing the reduction of health disparities
- Collecting and reporting data by race, ethnicity, preferred language, insurance, and SES

● Incorporating equity into the design and implementation of QI initiatives and evaluating whether interventions improve, sustain, or worsen disparities[1,6,18-21]

Quality improvement projects may worsen or maintain inequities if not explicitly evaluated. This potential for furthering inequities through QI and patient safety efforts underscores the need to collect, stratify, report, and display data by race, ethnicity, preferred language, insurance, and SES.[18,21] Figure 30–1 describes the possible impact of a QI project on disparities.[18] If data are not stratified by race, for example, combined outcomes may seem to improve and therefore conceal disparities (Figure 30–1a). Data stratified by race may reveal improvement for all groups with continued (Figure 30–1b), widened (Figure 30–1c), or narrowed (Figure 30–1d) disparities.[18]

Table 30–1. Applying an Equity Lens to Each Step of the Quality Improvement Process With Strategies for Equity-Focused Quality Improvement		
Steps in Improvement Frameworks[a,b]		**Strategies for Equity-Focused Quality Improvement[c,d,e–h]**
Define	What is our problem? What is our aim? What are we trying to accomplish? Who are our partners?	● Consider how disparities can be reduced through QI efforts.[e,h,i] ● Consider how the problem affects different populations. ● Identify disparities by stratifying existing quality measures, and prioritize the reduction of health disparities. ● Partner with QI analysts, disparities researchers, pediatric health professionals, patients and families, and communities to reduce disparities in care.

Table 30–1 (*continued*)		
Steps in Improvement Frameworks[a,b]		**Strategies for Equity-Focused Quality Improvement[c,d,e–h]**
Measure	How will we know that a change is an improvement?	● Collect data on race, ethnicity, preferred language, insurance, and socioeconomic status. Consider PROGRESS-Plus* variables.[j] Best practices include having patients self-identify rather than having an observer or team member assign race and ethnicity. ● Stratify and report data by race, ethnicity, and language preference. ● Be thoughtful when analyzing race-stratified data, and consider what the race variable is a proxy for describing. ● Identify disparities-sensitive measure(s) (eg, asthma-related emergency department visits, receipt of family-centered care, influenza immunization, pain management, hemoglobin A_{1c} testing, developmental screening, depression screening).[k] ● Display run charts and statistical process control charts stratified by race, ethnicity, and language preference data.
Analyze	What change can we make that will result in an improvement?	● Evaluate root causes, systems, and processes of disparities relevant to specific populations and the local environments. ● Incorporate equity into the design of QI initiatives (root cause analysis, key driver diagram, and study design, as well as metrics). ● Direct interventions to address disparities by focusing on populations with the greatest needs.
Improve	Implement change through Plan-Do-Study-Act cycles	● Normalize a culturally affirming approach to care, including implementing necessary tools, training, and staff time. ● Implement evidence-based interventions to reduce disparities. ● Evaluate whether interventions improve, sustain, or worsen disparities.

(continued on next page)

Table 30–1 (*continued*)		
Steps in Improvement Frameworks[a,b]		**Strategies for Equity-Focused Quality Improvement**[c,d,e–h]
Control	Sustain improvement	<ul><li>Ensure that leadership commitment, resources, and infrastructure are adequate and sustained.</li><li>Empower and equip quality officers to take on this work.</li></ul>

Abbreviation: QI, quality improvement.

* **P**lace of residence, **R**ace/ethnicity/culture/language, **O**ccupation, **G**ender/sex, **R**eligion, **E**ducation, **S**ocioeconomic status, **S**ocial capital, **P**lus other personal and relational features such as sexual orientation, disability, age, immigration status, and educational attainment.

[a] Langley GJ, Moen RD, Nolan KM, Nolan TW, Norman CL, Provost LP. *The Improvement Guide: A Practical Approach to Enhancing Organizational Performance.* 2nd ed. Jossey-Bass; 2009.

[b] George ML, Maxey J, Rowlands D, Price M, Maxey J. *The Lean Six Sigma Pocket Toolbook: A Quick Reference Guide to 100 Tools for Improving Quality and Speed.* McGraw-Hill; 2005.

[c] O'Kane M, Agrawal S, Binder L, et al. *An Equity Agenda for the Field of Health Care Quality Improvement.* National Academy of Medicine; 2021.

[d] Institute of Medicine Subcommittee on Standardized Collection of Race/Ethnicity Data for Healthcare Quality Improvement. *Race, Ethnicity, and Language Data: Standardization for Health Care Quality Improvement.* Ulmer C, McFadden B, Nerenz DR, eds. National Academies Press; 2009.

[e] Reichman V, Brachio SS, Madu CR, Montoya-Williams D, Peña MM. Using rising tides to lift all boats: Equity-Focused Quality Improvement as a tool to reduce neonatal health disparities. *Semin Fetal Neonatal Med.* 2021;26(1):101198.

[f] National Quality Forum. *A Road Map for Promoting Health Equity and Eliminating Disparities: The Four I's for Health Equity.* National Quality Forum; 2017.

[g] Lion KC, Raphael JL. Partnering health disparities research with quality improvement science in pediatrics. *Pediatrics.* 2015;135(2):354–361.

[h] Lion KC, Faro EZ, Coker TR. All quality improvement is health equity work: designing improvement to reduce disparities. *Pediatrics.* 2022;149(suppl 3):e2020045948E.

[i] Lau BD, Haider AH, Streiff MB, et al. Eliminating health care disparities with mandatory clinical decision support: the venous thromboembolism (VTE) example. *Med Care.* 2015;53(1):18–24.

[j] O'Neill J, Tabish H, Welch V, et al. Applying an equity lens to interventions: using PROGRESS ensures consideration of socially stratifying factors to illuminate inequities in health. *J Clin Epidemiol.* 2014;67(1):56–64.

[k] National Quality Forum. *Healthcare Disparities and Cultural Competency Consensus Standards: Disparities-Sensitive Measure Assessment.* National Quality Forum; 2012.

Figure 30-1. Potential Impact of a Quality Improvement Project on Disparities Between Populations, Highlighting the Importance of Stratifying Data

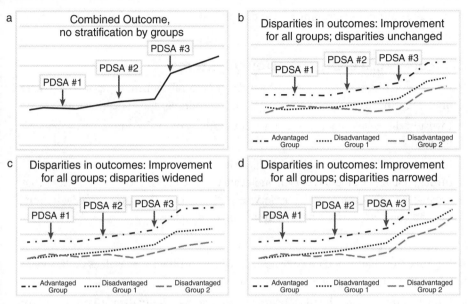

a, Combined outcomes for all populations with presumed improvement for all and no indication of disparities.
b–d, Disparities in stratified outcomes with improvement across groups, although disparities continue to be unchanged (b), widen (c), or narrow (d) over time. PDSA indicates Plan-Do-Study-Act.
Adapted with permission from Reichman V, Brachio SS, Madu CR, Montoya-Williams D, Peña MM. Using rising tides to lift all boats: Equity-Focused Quality Improvement as a tool to reduce neonatal health disparities. *Semin Fetal Neonatal Med.* 2021;26(1):101198.

Summary

There are many actions that pediatric health professional team members can take to further health equity through quality and safety efforts. We can

- Apply an equity lens across all aspects of quality and safety by assessing and measuring for disparities.
- Acknowledge, identify, and address disparities at the practice level by collecting, stratifying, and reporting data by race, ethnicity, and language preference.
- Use QI to focus on disparities and apply EF-QI principles at each step of the improvement process (Table 30-1).

Recommendations

Patient- and Family-Directed

- Engage patients and families as partners in QI and patient safety efforts.

- Foster trust in health care by increasing the quality of personal interactions, expanding workforce diversity, improving cultural and linguistic humility, and addressing implicit bias.
- Promote culturally representative and appropriate patient–pediatric health professional interactions.

Clinical Practice/Organizations/Systems

- Promote a culture of equity by normalizing a culturally affirming approach to care; implementing necessary tools, education, and training; and allocating time.
- Invest in the development, use, and accountability of health equity performance measures.[19]
- Incentivize the reduction of health disparities and achievement of health equity through payment model redesign and evaluation of economic impact. Ensure that organizations disproportionately serving individuals in under-resourced communities can compete in value-based purchasing programs.[19]

Measurement

- Improve the quality of data collected on race and ethnicity, as well as on language preference, insurance, SES, and other variables.
- Embed equity into quality dashboards to ensure that equity data are presented to health system leaders.
- Routinely stratify and report data by race and ethnicity to identify the greatest opportunities for improvement, set goals, and direct resources there.
- Update patient experience measures to include evaluation and accountability for the experience of bias and discrimination.

Leadership

- Ensure that leadership commitment, resources, and infrastructure are adequate and sustained.
- Ensure diverse leadership at all levels in quality and safety.
- Empower, equip, and fund quality officers within health care systems to take on this work.

Public Health Policy and Community Advocacy

- Advocate for strategies and resources to improve health literacy across populations.
- Advocate for funding to support the education and training of community health workers for their role in promoting health equity.
- Increase community involvement by cultivating formal and informal partnerships between community-based organizations and health systems and identifying resources to support these partnerships.

References

1. O'Kane M, Agrawal S, Binder L, et al. *An Equity Agenda for the Field of Health Care Quality Improvement.* National Academy of Medicine; 2021 doi: 10.31478/202109b
2. Institute of Medicine Committee on Quality of Health Care in America. *Crossing the Quality Chasm: A New Health System for the 21st Century.* National Academies Press; 2001:360
3. Institute of Medicine Committee on Future Directions for the National Healthcare Quality and Disparities Reports. *Future Directions for the National Healthcare Quality and Disparities Reports.* Ulmer C, Bruno M, Burke S, eds. National Academies Press; 2010
4. Institute of Medicine Committee on Understanding and Eliminating Racial and Ethnic Disparities in Health Care. *Unequal Treatment: Confronting Racial and Ethnic Disparities in Health Care.* Smedley BD, Stith AY, Nelson AR, eds. National Academies Press; 2003 PMID: 25032386
5. Institute of Medicine. *Toward Health Equity and Patient-Centeredness: Integrating Health Literacy Disparities Reduction, and Quality Improvement.* National Academies Press; 2009
6. Institute of Medicine Subcommittee on Standardized Collection of Race/Ethnicity Data for Healthcare Quality Improvement. *Race, Ethnicity, and Language Data: Standardization for Health Care Quality Improvement.* Ulmer C, McFadden B. Nerenz DR, eds. National Academies Press; 2009
7. Cowden JD, Flores G, Chow T, et al. Variability in collection and use of race/ethnicity and language data in 93 pediatric hospitals. *J Racial Ethn Health Disparities.* 2020;7(5):928–936 PMID: 32056162 doi: 10.1007/s40615-020-00716-8
8. Harrington R, Washington D, Paliani S, Thompson K, Rouse L, Anderson AC. A new effort to address racial and ethnic disparities in care through quality measurement. Health Affairs Forefront. September 9, 2021. Accessed June 7, 2023. https://www.healthaffairs.org/do/10.1377/forefront.20210907.568444/full
9. *2021 National Healthcare Quality and Disparities Report.* Agency for Healthcare Research and Quality; 2021. AHRQ publication 21(22)-0054-EF
10. Trent M, Dooley DG, Dougé J, et al; American Academy of Pediatrics Section on Adolescent Health, Council on Community Pediatrics, and Committee on Adolescence. The impact of racism on child and adolescent health. *Pediatrics.* 2019;144(2):e20191765 PMID: 31358665 doi: 10.1542/peds.2019-1765
11. Donabedian A. Evaluating the quality of medical care: 1966. *Milbank Q.* 2005;83(4):691–729 PMID: 16279964 doi: 10.1111/j.1468-0009.2005.00397.x
12. Wachter RM. *Understanding Patient Safety.* 3rd ed. McGraw-Hill; 2018
13. Frankel A, Haraden C, Federico F, Lenoci-Edwards J. *A Framework for Safe, Reliable, and Effective Care.* Institute for Healthcare Improvement and Safe & Reliable Healthcare; 2017
14. Chin MH. Advancing health equity in patient safety: a reckoning, challenge and opportunity. *BMJ Qual Saf.* 2020;bmjqs-2020–012599 PMID: 33376125 doi: 10.1136/bmjqs-2020-012599
15. Peek ME, Vela MB, Chin MH. Practical lessons for teaching about race and racism: successfully leading free, frank, and fearless discussions. *Acad Med.* 2020;95(12S):S139–S144 PMID: 32889939 doi: 10.1097/ACM.0000000000003710
16. Langley GJ, Moen RD, Nolan KM, Nolan TW, Norman CL, Provost LP. *The Improvement Guide: A Practical Approach to Enhancing Organizational Performance.* 2nd ed. Jossey-Bass; 2009
17. George ML, Rowlands D, Price M, Maxey J. *The Lean Six Sigma Pocket Toolbook: A Quick Reference Guide to 100 Tools for Improving Quality and Speed.* McGraw-Hill; 2005
18. Reichman V, Brachio SS, Madu CR, Montoya-Williams D, Peña MM. Using rising tides to lift all boats: Equity-Focused Quality Improvement as a tool to reduce neonatal health disparities. *Semin Fetal Neonatal Med.* 2021;26(1):101198 PMID: 33558160 doi: 10.1016/j.siny.2021.101198
19. National Quality Forum. *A Road Map for Promoting Health Equity and Eliminating Disparities: The Four I's for Health Equity.* National Quality Forum; 2017
20. Lion KC, Raphael JL. Partnering health disparities research with quality improvement science in pediatrics. *Pediatrics.* 2015;135(2):354–361 PMID: 25560436 doi: 10.1542/peds.2014-2982
21. Lion KC, Faro EZ, Coker TR. All quality improvement is health equity work: designing improvement to reduce disparities. *Pediatrics.* 2022;149(suppl 3):e2020045948E PMID: 35230431 doi: 10.1542/peds.2020-045948E

CHAPTER 31

Achieving Equity for Opportunity Youth

Kristin Mmari, DrPH, MA, and Vanya Jones, PhD, MPH

Who Are Opportunity Youth?

The term *opportunity youth* refers to youth who are between 16 and 24 years old, and because they are neither enrolled in school nor participating in the labor force, they are among the most difficult to serve youth communities for pediatric health professionals.[1] Previously referred to as *disconnected youth*, they compose a sizable proportion of youth in the United States. In 2019, right before the COVID-19 pandemic, there were more than 4.1 million opportunity youth in the United States, with disproportionate numbers among Native American, Black, Latinx,[a] and rural youth.[2] Despite a decade-long drop in the number of opportunity youth from 2011 to 2021, the number has now risen to more than 6 million because of economic downturns from the pandemic.[3]

Opportunity youth are not a homogenous group. Some left high school without a diploma, some experience no housing or transient housing, some have been involved in the youth legal system, and others are or were involved in foster care.[4] About half of opportunity youth have not been in school since the age of 16, whereas the other half have some schooling and work experience beyond the age of 16, including earning a high school diploma or GED.[4] Among female opportunity youth, motherhood rates are significantly higher than their connected counterparts experience: 25.2% versus 6%, respectively.[5] Overall, opportunity youth are more likely to live apart from their parents or caregivers, be from families with incomes below the federal poverty threshold, and lack health insurance.[6]

Experiencing disconnection during the critical period of emerging adulthood limits the chances and opportunities that youth will have throughout their lives. Youth who have been disconnected from school or work for at least 6 months are 3 times more likely to experience depression than youth who are connected to these key supports[1]; they are also one-sixth as likely to obtain a high school or college degree, a tendency hindering lifetime earnings, and are more likely to experience premature death from preventable conditions such as high blood pressure, diabetes, and stroke.[6] These individual costs are accompanied by a societal economic impact, with estimates ranging from $26.8 billion to $93 billion annually.[7]

---

[a] In this chapter, we use *Latinx* when referring to people of Latin Amerian origin or descent as a whole. It is a gender-neutral and gender-inclusive alternative to *Latino*. For a brief history of this term, including a rationale, refer to the book introduction.

To explore how to meet the needs of opportunity youth, this chapter focuses on

● Equity concerns that often disadvantage Black, Indigenous, and People of Color
● Institutional systems that contribute to youth becoming disconnected
● Opportunities for the health care system to engage with opportunity youth

Equity Concerns for Opportunity Youth

In the United States, Native American young men and boys experience the highest rate of disconnection (22.1%), followed by Native American young women and girls (20.8%) and Black young men and boys (19.5%).[8] The largest gender gap of any racial and ethnic group, Black young men and boys are significantly more likely to be disconnected than their female counterparts (13.7%). In contrast, only 9.2% of white youth are disconnected.[8]

In many ways, opportunity youth are like other adolescents and young adults growing up in a segregated society in the United States.[9] For example, Black American youth, on average, live in communities with few resources, poor housing quality, and overall higher environmental toxins that affect health and well-being.[10] Youth from predominately Black neighborhoods are often zoned to overcrowded and under-resourced schools.[11] Segregation in childhood and in early education exacerbates the disparities that Black, Indigenous, and Hispanic youth will face.[12] These disparities have fueled the narrative for how society portrays youth of color, particularly male youth of color, casting them as impulsive, hypermasculine, and impervious to social norms.[13] In addition, research has suggested that Black girls are treated more as adults, with less consideration for their developmental stages.[14] This *adultification* results in less guidance for and support of Black girls when compared to white girls experiencing trauma at the same ages.[14] These are damaging narratives and stereotypes that further perpetuate negative perceptions and treatment of Black youth.[13] They have also made us unaware about the role that institutions and policies have played in creating circumstances under which youth of color fail to thrive or are actively harmed.

Primary Institutional Systems With Critical Effects on Opportunity Youth

There are 4 primary institutional systems that have had critical effects on whether youth experience disconnection at some point in their lives: education, employment, child welfare, and juvenile justice/legal.[13]

Education

Among the most crucial resource deficiencies that many schools in segregated communities is the student to teacher ratio. Schools that serve high proportions of Black, Indigenous, and Hispanic youth have high ratios of students to teachers and a shortage of highly qualified teachers.[15] This deficiency affects the ability of schools to adequately serve students who are having difficulty and to offer opportunities for advanced classes to better prepare them for a college curriculum. Together with disproportionate suspensions/expulsions and school referrals to the youth legal system, these challenges can further disconnect youth of color, leading them to disengagement and even dropping out. The harsh, uneven enforcement of punishment as school disciplinary action for all Black students and the criminalization of loitering on school grounds when school is not in session, including policies such as "stop and frisk," increase the likelihood of incarceration for youth being on school property.[15,16]

Employment

Those who have received a poor education or lack trade skills face difficulty making a living wage. Yet, even with transferrable skills and knowledge, Black, Indigenous, and Hispanic youth still experience barriers, particularly if they live in segregated, limited-income neighborhoods or on Native American reservations. Black, Indigenous, and Hispanic youth often lack networks to link them with jobs or provide professional references. They are also likely not contacted because of their names and are deemed unprofessional when interviewing.[13] These factors illustrate how discrimination plays a significant role throughout the job application process.

Child Welfare System

It is well-known that there is an overrepresentation of children of color in the child welfare system relative to their representation in the general population. In 2019, Black children accounted for approximately 14% of the child population and 23% of the foster care system. That same year, white children made up half the child population and 44% of the foster care system.[17] These racial disparities in the child welfare system also fuel racial disparities among opportunity youth, particularly those who are "aging out" of the child welfare system. Several studies have shown that youth who age out of foster care have less stable employment and lower earnings than youth in the general population.[17]

Youth Legal System

Of all the systems discussed, the youth legal system has had the most devastating effect on the lives of youth of color. For example, boys and young men of color are subject to greater surveillance at a very early age, including at school.[18] When young men of color are charged with offenses, the legal system applies harsher sentences for them.[13,18] Although boys are more likely to be involved in the legal system, girls are more likely to experience arrest and enter the legal system for status offenses or noncriminal acts assigned only to minors, such as school truancy and running away from home.[14] Further, Black girls are more likely to be prosecuted for commercial/transactional sex, even though anyone younger than 18 years is protected as a youth who has been exploited through sex trafficking.[19] These types of arrests often lead to girls, mostly Black girls, experiencing increased legal system involvement over a lifetime for an offense that could have been better addressed via a child-centered developmental approach.[14] Because opportunity youth routinely fall prey to racist criminal justice/legal policies, reengaging them into education and employment systems will remain challenging unless there is dramatic system reform.

Summary

Unlike with youth connected to school systems, postsecondary institutions, and employers, there is no system or single point of contact through which opportunity youth are engaged and outcomes are measured. Opportunity youth need positive learning environments and resource networks to support their development, which will require supplemental supports from society such as providing mentors and considering an apprenticeship model as part of employment training. Health care is a key sector to focus on for opportunity youth. It accounts for 1 in 7 jobs in the US workforce.[20] In addition to building career pathways, pediatric health professionals are key in addressing the many needs and access to health services of opportunity youth. Policy makers, national experts, and researchers working to advance racial equity must address the needs of opportunity youth by taking bold steps to remove the numerous barriers they face.

Recommendations

Patient- and Family-Directed

- **Focus on mental health** because opportunity youth are in critical need of quality mental health and substance use/substance use disorder services, but they often do not have awareness of how to access help.
- **Connect eligible youth to public benefits** such as Medicaid and the Supplemental Nutrition Assistance Program to address health and food insecurity.

Clinical Practice/Organizations/Systems

- **Expand access to telehealth on both video and phone platforms** to reduce the barriers that youth face when seeking services.

Public Health Policy and Community Advocacy

- **Ensure that effective career pathways for opportunity youth** include advocating for[20]
  - *Implementing training and reinforcements* to address bias to eliminate the reduction in recruitment, interview, and job training.
  - *Creating work-friendly education opportunities* that make learning more accessible (eg, offering classes in the evening, on the weekends, and with adjustment to meet the needs of their schedules).

- *Ensuring there are learning-friendly* hospitals, nursing homes, and clinics to teach workers how to enter and learn jobs. Supervisors receive formal training to coach, mentor, and instruct workers in all work areas.

- *Fostering community-wide collaboration,* including pediatric health care professionals, high schools, colleges, other training professionals, and, possibly, organizations within the youth legal and child welfare systems, which often make up the infrastructure that underlies the career pathway in health for opportunity youth.

References

1. Mendelson T, Mmari K, Blum RW, Catalano RF, Brindis CD. Opportunity youth: insights and opportunities for a public health approach to reengage disconnected teenagers and young adults. *Public Health Rep.* 2018;133(suppl):54S–64S PMID: 30426873 doi: 10.1177/0033354918799344

2. Lewis K. *A Decade Undone: Youth Disconnection in the Age of Coronavirus.* Measure of America, Social Science Research Council; 2020. Accessed February 17, 2023. https://ssrc-static.s3.amazonaws.com/moa/ADecadeUndone.pdf

3. Miles M, Allen L. Working in partnership with opportunity youth. *Stanf Soc Innov Rev.* 2022 doi: 10.48558/0SQC-H806

4. Bridgeland J, Mason-Elder T. *National Roadmap for Opportunity Youth.* Civic Enterprises; 2012

5. Fernandes A, Gabe T. *Disconnected Youth: A Look at 16 to 24 Year Olds Who Are Not Working or in School.* US Congressional Research Service; 2015

6. Mendoza MJ. *After the Storm: Policy Recommendations to Reconnect Opportunity Youth During and After the COVID-19 Pandemic.* Aspen Institute Forum for Community Solutions; 2022

7. Lansford JE, Dodge KA, Pettit GS, Bates JE. A public health perspective on school dropout and adult outcomes: a prospective study of risk and protective factors from age 5 to 27 years. *J Adolesc Health.* 2016;58(6):652–658 PMID: 27009741 doi: 10.1016/j.jadohealth.2016.01.014

8. Lewis K. *A Decade Undone: 2021 Update.* Measure of America, Social Science Research Council; 2021. Accessed February 17, 2023. https://measureofamerica.org/youth-disconnection-2021

9. Acevedo-Garcia D, Lochner KA, Osypuk TL, Subramanian SV. Future directions in residential segregation and health research: a multilevel approach. *Am J Public Health.* 2003;93(2):215–221 PMID: 12554572 doi: 10.2105/AJPH.93.2.215

10. Bravo MA, Anthopolos R, Bell ML, Miranda ML. Racial isolation and exposure to airborne particulate matter and ozone in understudied US populations: environmental justice applications of downscaled numerical model output. *Environ Int.* 2016;92-93:247–255 PMID: 27115915 doi: 10.1016/j.envint.2016.04.008

11. Williams DR, Collins C. Racial residential segregation: a fundamental cause of racial disparities in health. *Public Health Rep.* 2001;116(5):404–416 PMID: 12042604 doi: 10.1016/S0033-3549(04)50068-7

12. Reskin B. The race discrimination system. *Annu Rev Sociol.* 2012;38(1):17–35 doi: 10.1146/annurev-soc-071811-145508

13. Rawlings LA. *Understanding the Environmental Contexts of Boys and Young Men of Color.* Urban Institute; 2015

14. Epstein R, Blake JJ, González T. *Girlhood Interrupted: The Erasure of Black Girls' Childhood.* Center of Poverty and Inequality, Georgetown Law; 2017

15. Office for Civil Rights. *Civil Rights Data Collection: Data Snapshot (Teacher Equity).* US Dept of Education; 2014

16. Fasching-Varner KJ, Mitchell RW, Martin LL, Bennett-Haron KP. Beyond school-to-prison pipeline and toward an educational and penal realism. *Equity Excell Educ.* 2014;47(4):410–429 doi: 10.1080/10665684.2014.959285

17. Child Welfare Information Gateway. *Child Welfare Practice to Address Racial Disproportionality and Disparity.* Children's Bureau, Administration for Children and Families, US Dept of Health and Human Services; 2021. Accessed February 17, 2023. https://www.childwelfare.gov/pubs/issue-briefs/racial-disproportionality

18. Kirk DS. Unraveling the contextual effects on student suspension and juvenile arrest: the independent and interdependent influences of school, neighborhood, and family social controls. *Criminology.* 2009;47(2):479–520 doi: 10.1111/j.1745-9125.2009.00147.x

19. Brooks S. Innocent white victims and fallen Black girls: race, sex work, and the limits of anti-sex trafficking laws. *Signs (Chic Ill).* 2021;46(2):513–515 doi: 10.1086/710816

20. Wilson R. *Health Care Pathways for Opportunity Youth: A Framework for Practitioners and Policymakers.* Jobs for the Future, California Endowment; 2014

CHAPTER 32

Pediatric and Adolescent Research on Race and Racism

Tamera Coyne-Beasley, MD, MPH, and María Verónica Svetaz, MD, MPH

"Race" and "ethnicity" are poorly defined terms that serve as flawed surrogates for multiple environmental and genetic factors in disease causation, including ancestral geographic origins, socioeconomic status, education, and access to health care. Research must move beyond these weak and imperfect proxy relationships to define the more proximate factors that influence health.

Francis S. Collins, MD, PhD, former director, National Institutes of Health and Human Genome Project[1]

Introduction

The increase in hate crimes over the past decade combined with centuries of social and racial injustice have catalyzed an urgency for scientists to examine what we, the authors, describe as the *racism research gap*: the unacceptable lack of research on effective interventions and best practices to promote resiliency and address racism as a social determinant of health (SDOH), an adverse childhood experience (ACE), and a source of chronic stress among children and adolescents.[2] Although research has advanced to identify and understand some impacts of race and racism, there remain significant gaps in evidence-based interventions about dismantling and mitigating its effects, including the resultant health disparities in and adverse effects on child and adolescent development.[3]

What Do We Know About Race?

Race is a social construct created to classify and categorize people, create hierarchies, and ensure unequal distribution of privilege, resources, freedom, and power. Data from the National Human Genome Research Institute reveal that although an individual may have more than 3 million differences in their genome compared with someone else's, humans share 99.9% of the same DNA.[4] The differences people observe (eg, skin color, hair texture, bone structure) are known as *clines*, which do not qualify humans to be distinguished into different biological races. Race only minimally describes biologically or genetically distinct groups and is a social concept, not a scientific one. The United

Nations Educational, Scientific and Cultural Organization 1950 statement on race included this incisive affirmation: "race is less a biological fact than a social myth and as a myth it has taken a heavy toll in human lives and suffering."[5]

What Do We Know About Racism?

Racism has significant and often catastrophic biological and multigenerational consequences that lead to health disparities. Children and adolescents exposed to racial discrimination (personally or vicariously) at the individual, peer/family/community, institutional, and societal levels experience profound effects on their psychological and biological functioning (Table 32–1).

How Has Race Been Misused?

Within race-based medicine, misuse of race as an already flawed concept is notable. In this circumstance, race is used as a proxy for genetic ancestry or epigenetics in clinical decision-making or the research that drives innovation. One example is the now-retired "Urinary Tract Infection: Clinical Practice Guideline for the Diagnosis and Management of the Initial UTI in Febrile Infants and Children 2 to 24 Months."[6] In this case, race was inappropriately inserted as a default biological proxy in lieu of incompletely explained epidemiological observation. The scientific community must dismantle and replace clinical practice guidelines that use race as an independent risk-adjusting variable. In the absence of more definitive science, the just approach is to confer equitable care to all children regardless of race.[7] Race has also been misused in science to claim superiority and to justify racial discrimination and the exclusionary, inequitable treatment of specific ethnic groups.[8]

Why Do We Still Need to Measure Race?

Balanced scientific discourse has argued that even with insurmountable evidence to support that race is not a direct proxy for genetic difference, there is still a role for what race represents in accounting for differential lived experiences and exposures. Using scientific integrity and rigorously sorting the social and political determinants or influencers of health are critical for transformative discovery to which scientists must be accountable.[7] We must also remove the "minority" status and the collective minority categorization of people of color; they are inaccurate, nonscientific, obsolete, and hierarchal. Scientific language should not stigmatize or reproduce oppressive forms of power.[9]

How Has Race Been Measured?

Research on race and racism has been limited by the categorical, variable measures of race and ethnicity that are based on perceived phenotype. Additionally, the measures of race and ethnicity often do not account for the significant heterogeneity found within

Table 32–1. Select Effects of Racial Discrimination on Children and Adolescents	
Level of Exposure	**Effects on Psychological and Biological Functioning**
Individual	● Adverse cognitive and emotional processes and associated psychopathological processes ● Diminished participation in healthy behaviors (eg, sleep and exercise) ● Increased engagement in unhealthy behaviors (eg, alcohol consumption) either directly, as stress coping, or indirectly, via reduced self-regulation ● Concomitant pathophysiological processes, or the increases in allostatic load and stress that grind down on the body in multiple unhealthy modalities, affecting the individual's brain, immune system, and inflammatory response ● Altered physiological functioning ● Heightened perceptions of threat, fear, or victimization ● Low self-efficacy, low self-esteem, and hopelessness ● Increased internalizing behaviors (eg, depression, anxiety, and isolation) ● Increased externalizing behaviors (eg, aggression and violence) ● Physical injury caused by racist violence ● Death
Family	● Negative youth outcomes and experience with racism also affect the health and well-being of parents, caregivers, and extended family and may reduce their capacity to shield, and enhance the lives of, their children and adolescents.
Transgenerational	● The stress of racism causes DNA changes in which the impacts of racism can be transmitted transgenerationally and can lead to serious physical illnesses and mental health conditions. ● Epigenetics, or the interaction of genes, stress, and environment, can lead to altered DNA or associated proteins that, although they do not change the actual coding sequence of DNA, may affect DNA function.

groups such as Latine[a] groups, which include individuals from the Caribbean, Central America and South America, and Spain. Further, the sample size of many populations that have been racialized often does not meet statistical significance to make any specific inferences about race. The measure of race has more to do with group similarities in experience with bias and discrimination than the inherent color of one's skin or the behavior of an individual or a group.

A recent compendium measuring race and ethnicity has gathered a focused collection of instruments using race or ethnicity.[10] Most previous efforts have focused on a single racial or ethnic group or have primarily addressed either health/mental health issues or identity concerns. This volume focuses on intra- and inter-social psychological measures across several racial and ethnic groups. The authors have focused on white, Hispanic, Native American, Asian American and Pacific Islander, and African American groups and their perceptions of self and interactions with others. It is evident from the instruments listed that scale development for some racial and ethnic groups, such as Native American groups, is sorely needed.

How Should We Use Race?

The use of race should be limited to monitor health inequities. Health inequities are rooted in the unequal distribution of the aforementioned SDOH. Researchers should aspire to measure root causes of disease, moving away from weakly correlated variables, such as self-identified race or ethnicity, toward an understanding of the more proximate environmental and genetic factors.[1] To measure environmental factors means using an ecological approach to research design. Acknowledging and measuring social determinants is critical when they contribute to the deleterious health outcomes disproportionately borne by communities that have been marginalized through structural policies that create unequal distribution of assets and opportunities. So is measuring the higher stress in these communities caused by the constant lifelong effect of bias, discrimination, and stereotyping.[11] This framework needs to be universally included in research designed to explore health equities and community health. The "expanded" ACEs[12] are an example; they include adverse community environments and adverse cultural exposures. Because individuals can have multiple marginalized identities, research grounded in intersectionality increasingly underscores that multiple marginalizing social categories intersect to amplify health inequities.[13] Research on race and racism needs to include measurements of SDOH, ACEs, and intersectionality to get to the root of the effect of environmental and genetic factors.

The researcher and research consumer should have race consciousness.[14] This concept encompasses

- Deep awareness of one's racial position through self-exploration and critical consciousness

---

[a] In this chapter, we use *Latine* when referring to people of Latin American origin or descent as a whole. It is a gender-neutral and gender-inclusive alternative to *Latino*. For a brief history of this term, including a rationale, refer to the book introduction.

- Awareness of the racial stratification processes that were and are operating in racial-neutral contexts (also called *color-evasive contexts*), plus the understanding that historical research tended to attribute effects to race rather than to racialization or racism

- Eradication of biological determinism, or the belief that race is meaningful because it provides insights about one's biology and propensities

Summary

Scientific research will be critical for developing evidence-based effective interventions to mitigate the impacts of racism and its resultant health disparities. More importantly, dismantling racism will require a comprehensive, multi-sector, interdisciplinary, and life course approach across all levels of the socio-ecological framework with a focus on the SDOH. It is our role and responsibility as research scientists and scientific consumers to reimagine and work toward creating a world without racism. This may include collecting necessary data; implementing evidence-based strategies in clinical care; advocating for anti-racist policies, practices, and programs; and leveraging research funding to evaluate racism alongside the biological markers of disease or clinical outcomes. Simply abandoning the term *race* without rectifying the disparities denoted by this poor proxy for social status and generational inequity will allow the cycle of trauma to continue across generations of children, adolescents, and families and prevent them from achieving healthy and bright futures.

The need to generate new research about race and racism on health outcomes is urgent. We hope the tables provided in this chapter create awareness of the impact of racism on different health outcomes, provide resources for how to measure racism in research, and summarize main recommendations by national institutions and organizations on the next steps.

Recommendations

Patient- and Family-Directed

- Document SDOH related to clinical outcomes.
- Allow patients and families to report their socially assigned races and their self-identified races.[15]
- Assess for racial and ethnic discrimination (Table 32–2).

Public Health Policy and Community Advocacy

- Incorporate the following data into intervention development and evaluation:
  - Area-level social risk factors from US Census data or the American Community Survey to reflect data at the neighborhood level

- Composite measures from these data: Area Deprivation Index (ADI), Social Vulnerability Index (SVI), and Child Opportunity Index (COI)

Interventions are needed at all levels of the socio-ecological framework, including the societal levels. Table 32–3 summarizes recommended research and efforts needed as identified by national organizations and institutions. Research funding is also critically important to evaluate the role of race and racism on health outcomes and the subsequent use of race and racism in research. Part of an anti-racism commitment is that each of us must hold ourselves, our colleagues, institutions, organizations, and society accountable for the design, conduct, and implementation of research that adheres to the principles and recommendations outlined by our professional organizations to reduce racial inequities in child and adolescent health.

| Table 32–2. Select Instruments to Measure Racial Discrimination ||
Domains	Instrument(s)
Racial and ethnic discrimination	● Everyday Discrimination Scale (EDS) ● Child Perceived Discrimination Questionnaire (CPDQ) ● Perceptions of Racism in Children and Youth (PRaCY) ● Daily Life Experiences—Frequency Scale (DLE-F) ● Racism Experiences Stress Scale (EXP-STR) ● Index of Race-Related Stress (IRRS) ● Adolescent Discrimination Distress Index (ADDI) ● Hispanic Stress Inventory—Adolescent Version (HSI-A)
Acculturative stress	● Social, Attitudinal, Familial, and Environmental Acculturative Stress Scale for Children (SAFE-C) ● Acculturative Stress Inventory for Children (ASIC)
Bicultural stress	● Mexican American Biculturalism Scale (MABS)

Table 32–3. Summary of Additional Race and Racism Research Needs Recommended by Select National Organizations to Reduce Inequities	
National Organization	**Research Needs Recommended**
The **American Academy of Pediatrics** recommends research to examine	• The impact of perceived and observed experiences of discrimination on child and family health outcomes • The role of self-identification over perceived race on child health access, status, and outcomes • The impact of workforce-development activities on patient satisfaction, trust, care use, and pediatric health outcomes • The impact of policy changes and community-level interventions on reducing the health effects of racism and other forms of discrimination on youth development • The integration of the human genome as a way to identify critical biomarkers that can be used to improve human health rather than to continue to classify people on the basis of their minor genetic differences and their countries of origin
The **American Psychological Association** recommends research to examine	• How to address racism for perpetrators of racism • Identity development and interaction with critical consciousness • Protective interventions that foster a positive cultural (racial and ethnic) identity • Protective interventions that prevent the internalization of racism

(continued on next page)

Table 32–3 (*continued*)	
National Organization	**Research Needs Recommended**
The **Centers for Disease Control and Prevention** CORE Health Equity and Science Intervention Strategy includes efforts to	● **C**ultivate comprehensive health equity science; embed health equity principles within the design, implementation, and evaluation of research, data, and surveillance in intervention strategies. ● **O**ptimize interventions by using scientific, innovative, and data-driven intervention strategies to address environmental, place-based, occupational, policy, and system factors that affect health outcomes and to address drivers of health disparities. ● **R**einforce and expand robust partnerships: multilevel, multi-sectoral, and community partnerships. ● **E**nhance capacity and workforce engagement by cultivating a multidisciplinary workforce and more inclusive climates, policies, and practices for broader public health impact.
The **National Institutes of Health** Diversity, Equity, Inclusion, and Accessibility Strategic Plan; UNITE initiative; and Chief Officer for Scientific Workforce Diversity Strategic Plan include	● Actions to increase diversity in biomedical workforces, particularly at leadership levels, and to decrease funding discrepancies among grantees ● Actions to increase funding to support research initiatives and improve monitoring and program evaluation • For example, the NIH Common Fund Transformative Research to Address Health Disparities and Advance Health Equity initiative has committed up to $58 million for these efforts. ● A multifaceted approach that reviews and modifies NIH policies, processes, practices, and cultural norms while ensuring accountability, sustainability, and transparency

Table 32–3 (*continued*)	
National Organization	**Research Needs Recommended**
The **Robert Wood Johnson Foundation** recommends	● Developing a robust, modern data infrastructure that collects data between public health and other sectors: housing, education, employment, and other SDOH ● Improving the collection of self-reported data by race, other SDOH, and intersectionality ● Developing powerful local data collaboratives to link SDOH that are now missing in most governmental public health data sets to enable local health departments in partnership with community organizations to prioritize and address local health challenges ● Building community-academic partnerships with historically Black colleges and universities to expand capacity in the creation, collection, analysis, and interpretation of data
The **Society for Adolescent Health and Medicine** recommends[a]	● Research on effective interventions and best practices to promote resiliency and address racism, chronic stress, and vicarious trauma affecting youth, trainees, and youth-serving professionals of color. Individual- and societal-level interventions are necessary. ● Community-engaged, participatory, and life course research approaches to develop, implement, and evaluate policies, processes, and practices and decolonize research. ● Pediatric health professionals caring for youth should develop research and integrate promising interventions to address racism as part of routine evaluation and in response to identified aggression.

Abbreviations: NIH, National Institutes of Health; SDOH, social determinants of health.

[a] Racism and its harmful effects on nondominant racial–ethnic youth and youth-serving providers: a call to action for organizational change: the Society for Adolescent Health and Medicine. *J Adolesc Health*. 2018;63(2):257–261.

References

1. Collins FS. What we do and don't know about 'race', 'ethnicity', genetics and health at the dawn of the genome era. *Nat Genet.* 2004;36(11)(suppl):S13–S15 PMID: 15507997 doi: 10.1038/ng1436

2. Racism and its harmful effects on nondominant racial–ethnic youth and youth-serving providers: a call to action for organizational change: the Society for Adolescent Health and Medicine. *J Adolesc Health.* 2018;63(2):257–261 PMID: 30149927 doi: 10.1016/j.jadohealth.2018.06.003

3. Miller MJ, Keum BT, Thai CJ, et al. Practice recommendations for addressing racism: a content analysis of the counseling psychology literature. *J Couns Psychol.* 2018;65(6):669–680 PMID: 30091623 doi: 10.1037/cou0000306

4. Collins FS, Mansoura MK. The Human Genome Project: revealing the shared inheritance of all humankind. *Cancer.* 2001;91(1)(suppl):221–225 PMID: 11148583 doi: 10.1002/1097-0142(20010101)91:1+<221::AID-CNCR8>3.0.CO;2-9

5. UNESCO launches major world campaign against racial discrimination. In: *Statement on Race - Part I.* United Nations Educational, Scientific and Cultural Organization; 1950:208–210. File 323.12 A 102. Accessed February 20, 2023. https://atom.archives.unesco.org

6. Kowalsky RH, Rondini AC, Platt SL. The case for removing race from the American Academy of Pediatrics clinical practice guideline for urinary tract infection in infants and young children with fever. *JAMA Pediatr.* 2020;174(3):229–230 PMID: 31930353 doi: 10.1001/jamapediatrics.2019.5242

7. Wright JL, Freed GL, Hendricks-Muñoz KD, et al; Committee on Diversity, Inclusion and Equity on behalf of the American Pediatric Society. Achieving equity through science and integrity: dismantling race-based medicine. *Pediatr Res.* 2022;91(7):1641–1644 PMID: 35383261 doi: 10.1038/s41390-022-02041-84

8. Tucker WH. The ideology of racism: misusing science to justify racial discrimination. *UN Chronicle.* Accessed February 20, 2023. https://www.un.org/en/chronicle/article/ideology-racism-misusing-science-justify-racial-discrimination

9. Corneau S, Stergiopoulos V. More than being against it: anti-racism and anti-oppression in mental health services. *Transcult Psychiatry.* 2012;49(2):261–282 PMID: 22508637 doi: 10.1177/1363461512441594

10. Davis LE, Engel RJ. *Measuring Race and Ethnicity.* Springer Science+Business Media; 2011 doi: 10.1007/978-1-4419-6697-1

11. Sapolsky RM. The health-wealth gap. *Sci Am.* 2018;319(5):62–67 PMID: 30328837 doi: 10.1038/scientificamerican1118-62

12. Cronholm PF, Forke CM, Wade R, et al. Adverse childhood experiences: expanding the concept of adversity. *Am J Prev Med.* 2015;49(3):354–361 PMID: 26296440 doi: 10.1016/j.amepre.2015.02.001

13. Khan M, Ilcisin M, Saxton K. Multifactorial discrimination as a fundamental cause of mental health inequities. *Int J Equity Health.* 2017;16(1):43 PMID: 28257630 doi: 10.1186/s12939-017-0532-z

14. Ford CL, Airhihenbuwa CO. The public health critical race methodology: praxis for antiracism research. *Soc Sci Med.* 2010;71(8):1390–1398 PMID: 20822840 doi: 10.1016/j.socscimed.2010.07.030

15. Jones CP, Truman BI, Elam-Evans LD, et al. Using "socially assigned race" to probe white advantages in health status. *Ethn Dis.* 2008;18(4):496–504 PMID: 19157256

Part 3. Optimizing Anti-racism in Practice

Section 3. Public Health, Policy, and Advocacy

CHAPTER 33

Child Health Advocacy and Anti-racism

Jean L. Raphael, MD, MPH, and Lee Savio Beers, MD

Introduction

Since the publication of the Institute of Medicine report *Unequal Treatment: Confronting Racial and Ethnic Disparities in Health Care*,[1] inequities in the United States health care system have received unprecedented attention from clinicians, researchers, and policy makers. Over time, this focus has expanded to include upstream drivers of health as goals of advocacy efforts both within the health care system and in society at large. Although this comprehensive approach has elevated the discourse on the root causes of inequities, it has failed to acknowledge the overarching and crosscutting role of structural racism in undermining child health.[2] Increasing recognition of racism as a public health crisis has brought a new understanding of the historical context of the communities that have been marginalized and the policies (eg, redlining, gentrification, mass incarceration) that have been implemented by policy makers and have led to racial injustice.[2,3] It has also demonstrated health care as a perpetrator of racism in both care delivery and research, with resultant mistrust on the part of children, adolescents, and families.

As pediatric health professionals embrace the necessary work of dismantling racism in medical education, clinical care, and research, they must also adopt new principles and strategies in child health advocacy. This chapter provides an overview of child health advocacy, discusses advocacy as a professional standard, and outlines how to engage in advocacy centered on anti-racism. Although the focus of this chapter is on pediatric health professionals, the content of it is also relevant to other youth-serving allied health professionals, team members, and collaborators.

Overview of Advocacy

Advocacy represents "action by a physician to promote those social, economic, educational, and political changes that ameliorate the suffering and threats to human health and well-being." It has been a critical component of pediatrics since its inception and an essential component in the formation of the American Academy of Pediatrics.[4] Although pediatric health professionals understand their role as advocates for individual patients in clinical settings, they may be less knowledgeable in the constructs of systems-directed advocacy that require addressing the root causes of the problems families encounter. The spectrum of systems-directed advocacy occurs at several levels. Pediatric health professionals may engage in *organization-level* advocacy in which the goals of efforts exist within a practice, hospital, or health care organization.

Such anti-racism advocacy efforts may include removing race from clinical algorithms, addressing inequities in security calls against families, and promoting language inclusivity. Outside of practice settings, pediatric health professionals may participate in *community-level advocacy* in which the focus is an issue that affects a local community. Anti-racism advocacy may focus on creating healthful food markets, improving education quality, or sustaining green spaces in under-resourced or segregated communities. Last, pediatric health professionals may engage in *government-level advocacy* (ie, local, state, federal) in which the goal is to influence regulatory and budgetary policies. Such anti-racism efforts may include advocacy for alternative strategies to incarceration, appropriation of mental health resources, and fair practices in housing.

Advocacy as a Professional Standard

Perhaps because of its particular focus on the developmental life course, pediatrics has been a leader within medicine in addressing social influences on health.[4] Yet this commitment has not been without challenge or controversy. There has been historical debate over the role of the physician in advocacy, emphasizing the need to remain unbiased and nonpartisan: a significant challenge that is heightened in a politically divisive environment.[4] Regardless, there has been increasing consensus by medical organizations that advocacy is an essential professional competency.[4] A recent survey of pediatric program directors showed that 80% of respondents thought that advocacy was more important within their academic departments than 5 years prior and an equal percentage thought that advocacy would be "more" or "much more" important in the future.[5]

Advocacy Strategies

Central to advocacy is the need for action, which can be formulated and implemented in many ways to achieve overall policy objectives.

- *Media advocacy* represents a mechanism to increase public awareness, interact with a broad range of stakeholders, and influence decision-makers through targeted mass media outlets. Examples include newspaper and radio stories, op-eds, press conferences, and social media posts. Media advocacy requires concise and compelling messaging (eg, sound bites, visual images, data).

- *Education-based advocacy* consists of actions to increase overall knowledge on a specific topic. Examples include issue briefs, policy briefs, seminars, and conferences.

- *Legislative advocacy* comprises synergistic efforts to influence introduction, enactment, or modification of legislation. The most common means of legislative advocacy is direct engagement or long-term strategic partnership with a legislative office to share views on an issue and request a specific action or vote. This interaction may involve letter writing, phone calls, or formal meetings. Legislative testimony provides another tool by which to participate in legislative advocacy.

Pediatric health professionals have numerous avenues to apply these strategies on behalf of a larger organization, such as a health system, professional society, or non-profit, or as individuals.[4,6] Understanding the strengths and limitations of these different approaches can help guide advocacy efforts. When working on behalf of an organization, it is critical to ensure that advocacy activities are consistent with the organization's positions on a particular issue. Misaligned or lacking communication can lead to confusion and conflicting messages, ultimately undermining advocacy efforts. Although the weight and resources of an institution can add strength to advocacy efforts, its policy positions are typically influenced by the breadth of activities it engages in and the overall policy environment, which may lead to de-prioritization of otherwise essential issues. Additionally, the pace of change may be slower given potentially competing influences. An individual advocating on their own behalf has more autonomy and can act more nimbly, but they usually do not have similar resources available. One approach to address this tension is to work with community organizations; an added strength to this approach may include shared learning and a closer alignment with those who are more directly affected by an issue.[3] This is particularly relevant when advocating for issues such as the effect of racism on child health, in which individuals' lived experiences vary widely and there has been prolonged and systemic oppression of a group of people.

Engaging in Advocacy Centered in Anti-racism

Complex challenges require a multidisciplinary and collaborative approach and can be strengthened by partnerships within and outside the health system. Authentic and substantive engagement of people most affected (eg, families, caregivers, and community members) is an essential strategy to ground advocacy in anti-racist principles. The expert leadership of professionals working on health equity throughout their careers should also be included and elevated. This sharing of power and centering of community voice often require a different approach than is typical in health systems, with additional competencies needed that are related to the values and best practices of community engagement.[3,7] Other partners may also include professionals or organizations such as medical professional societies, government affairs specialists, family-run organizations, legal advocacy groups, government leaders, and researchers.[4] Coordinating multidisciplinary collaborations is likely beyond the scope of most individual pediatric health professionals. But they can play an essential role as contributors to existing efforts.

Although there are many facilitators of engagement, pediatric health professionals also face numerous barriers to engaging in advocacy focused on anti-racism and the impact of racism on child health. These barriers often center around time, resources, competing priorities, workforce diversity, and political climate.[3] For academicians, challenges include integrating advocacy activities into teaching and scholarship.[6] Additionally, child health advocates face hostility and public attacks or threats, both online and in person.

Summary

As pediatric health professionals increasingly apply an anti-racist framework to clinical care, research, and education, it is paramount that this approach becomes rooted in advocacy. Being effective advocates for dismantling racism requires modernizing our concept of professional standards, understanding the full breadth of advocacy strategies, and tailoring our engagement to be goal driven and collaborative with the communities we aspire to empower.

Recommendations

Patient- and Family-Directed

● Empower families to advocate for themselves and their communities.

Clinical Practice/Organizations/Systems

● Identify available time and resources. Sometimes these supports can be made available by realigning existing activities or funds or by looking to external partnerships. Medical professional societies such as the American Academy of Pediatrics are an important resource.

● For professionals working in academic medicine, consider developing an advocacy portfolio to integrate your advocacy into your scholarly activities, support your personal career development, and contribute to learning within the field.[6]

Public Health Policy and Community Advocacy

● Commit to ongoing individual learning with adequate time, introspection, and humility. A knowledge of historical injustice and the impact of racism on current-day systems is essential to understand and responsibly address the effects of racism on child health.

● Identify mentors, peer supports, and champions. Care should be taken to ensure that these relationships are mutually supportive and beneficial, particularly for individuals from groups that are underrepresented in medicine and therefore often overburdened with requests for related consultation or assistance.

● Set both short- and long-term goals with tangible milestones. Sometimes it can be helpful to "start small" to build and strengthen your relationships, hone your skills, and better understand your working environment before tackling larger initiatives.

● Consider additional training. Successful advocacy requires a specific set of skills and experiences that can be cultivated and strengthened through formal learning opportunities.

References

1. Institute of Medicine Committee on Understanding and Eliminating Racial and Ethnic Disparities in Health Care. *Unequal Treatment: Confronting Racial and Ethnic Disparities in Health Care.* Smedley BD, Stith AY, Nelson AR, eds. National Academies Press; 2003

2. Heard-Garris N, Boyd R, Kan K, Perez-Cardona L, Heard NJ, Johnson TJ. Structuring poverty: how racism shapes child poverty and child and adolescent health. *Acad Pediatr.* 2021;21(8)(suppl):S108–S116 PMID: 34740417 doi: 10.1016/j.acap.2021.05.026

3. Trent M, Dooley DG, Dougé J, et al; American Academy of Pediatrics Section on Adolescent Health, Council on Community Pediatrics, and Committee on Adolescence. The impact of racism on child and adolescent health. *Pediatrics.* 2019;144(2):e20191765 PMID: 31358665 doi: 10.1542/peds.2019-1765

4. Shah SI, Brumberg HL. Advocating for advocacy in pediatrics: supporting lifelong career trajectories. *Pediatrics.* 2014;134(6):e1523–e1527 PMID: 25422021 doi: 10.1542/peds.2014-0211

5. Chung RJ, Ramirez MR, Best DL, Cohen MB, Chamberlain LJ. Advocacy and community engagement: perspectives from pediatric department chairs. *J Pediatr.* 2022;248:6–10.e3 PMID: 35032554 doi: 10.1016/j.jpeds.2021.12.019

6. Nerlinger AL, Shah AN, Beck AF, et al. The advocacy portfolio: a standardized tool for documenting physician advocacy. *Acad Med.* 2018;93(6):860–868 PMID: 29298182 doi: 10.1097/ACM.0000000000002122

7. Alberti P, Fair M, Skorton DJ. Now is our time to act: why academic medicine must embrace community collaboration as its fourth mission. *Acad Med.* 2021;96(11):1503–1506 PMID: 34432717 doi: 10.1097/ACM.0000000000004371

CHAPTER 34

Public Health: Disparities and Inequities in Your Community

Joshua M. Sharfstein, MD, and Michelle Spencer, MS

Introduction

On September 24, 2015, pediatrician Mona Hanna-Attisha, MD, MPH, FAAP, called a press conference.[1] Her research, published that same day in the *American Journal of Public Health*,[2] had identified a clear connection between the water supply of Flint, MI, and rising lead levels in the city's children. Her words to the media demanded action: "We are advocating for a switch back to a Lake Huron water source.... [There is] no safe level of lead for a child."[3]

The press conference revealed an outrageous act of environmental racism: the switching of a city's water to save money without the engagement of its residents and the ignoring of multiple concerns about its smell, color, taste, and clarity. Dr Hanna-Attisha would later say, "This never would have happened in a richer or whiter community."[4] Flint residents heard their local pediatrician speak the truth. Not long afterward, despite many attempts to dismiss her, the state of Michigan listened too and changed the city's water supply. The Obama administration paid attention, mobilizing multiple agencies to support programs for children in Flint.[5] Eventually, even Congress took action, providing billions of dollars to remove lead pipes across the country.[6] Dr Hanna-Attisha's extraordinary success illustrates the power that pediatric health professionals have when they draw attention to the impact of racism and to the inequities in their own communities.

Pediatric health professionals are uniquely positioned to explain 2 fundamental insights: child and adolescent health depends on a safe physical and social environment, and this environment has been warped by racism. A few specific examples of the resulting inequities include

- **Toxic exposures.** In addition to experiencing tainted water supplies, Black children, Hispanic children, and children in limited-income settings are also more likely to breathe in polluted air and come into contact with polluted soil.

- **Educational quality.** Black, Hispanic, and Indigenous children and adolescents are less likely to attend schools with a full range of math and science courses and extra-curricular activities.[7]

- **Economic opportunities.** Black, Hispanic, and Indigenous adolescents and young adults are less likely to be employed than white adolescents and young adults and are more likely to be disconnected from both school and employment.[8]

- **Policing.** Policing abuses disproportionately and deleteriously affect the physical and mental health of Black adolescents.[9]

In 1988, the Institute of Medicine defined public health as "what…society [does] collectively to assure the conditions for people to be healthy."[10] Beyond providing high-quality patient care, pediatric health professionals can engage in their communities to counter the structures of racism and improve the conditions of health. Critical roles for pediatric health professionals include identifying and analyzing racial inequities at the community level and then developing and advocating for solutions.

Identifying and Analyzing Racial Inequities

Sometimes, critical data on community health disparities are situated right in the pediatric clinic files. Dr Hanna-Attisha's pivotal analysis drew on her hospital's lead-poisoning records. Other important data sources include the records of coroners or medical examiners, as well as state and local vital statistics reports, which contain data on infant death and low birth weight by race and ethnicity. Pediatric health professionals can search data from national surveys, such as those on nutrition, addiction, and health behaviors. Busy pediatric health professionals should consider reaching out to local public health schools to find graduate students, often with requirements for practicum experiences, as well as faculty interested in collaborating.

With data in hand, the next step is analysis. Dr Hanna-Attisha worked with statisticians and geographers at Michigan State University to identify a dose response as an indicator of causality; the children with the greatest exposure to Flint water had the highest levels of lead. Her findings, and their publication in a prestigious journal, eventually overcame the fierce objections and personal attacks by state officials.

There are other techniques in data analysis that may also help pediatric health professionals. Visualizing the impact of school conditions on the attendance and health of children and adolescents in Baltimore helped generate support for new infrastructure investments.[11] Extrapolating from small samples to large populations allowed pediatric residents in Boston to call attention to the impact of housing conditions on child and adolescent health outcomes.[12]

Developing and Advocating for Solutions

Understanding inequities puts pediatric health professionals in a position to develop an agenda for change. These solutions can include programs, which are specific efforts tailored to discrete populations, and policies, which change the way that governments and the private sector operate. It is possible to combine immediate and long-term steps into an agenda for change. In Flint, MI, for example, Dr Hanna-Attisha not only called for an urgent change in the water supply but also advocated for a removal of lead pipes across the city, an investment in early childhood education, and other, more fundamental reforms.

A common question is how to find the right solutions to a particular problem. Pediatric health professionals are likely familiar with the African proverb that it takes a village to raise a child, popularized by Hillary Clinton in her vision for the children of America. A parallel concept is that it takes a community to solve complicated challenges. Pediatric health professionals can reach out to local lawyers and policy experts to understand the policy history and landscape, including active proposals under consideration. Simultaneously, they can listen to the ideas of their patients and their families. Many may already be participating in coalitions that have developed detailed agendas, such as the adolescent-led March For Our Lives campaign against gun violence, the parent-led Mothers Against Drunk Driving, and efforts to overturn misinformed laws on what can be taught in classrooms on race or gender identity. These coalitions can connect with other groups at the state and national levels for even greater impact.

Pediatric health professionals can play different roles in advocacy efforts. One approach, used by Dr Hanna-Attisha, is to call reporters for a press conference. Other options include issuing a report, writing a letter to journalists, publishing a scientific commentary, or writing for a local or national newspaper. For example, pediatrician Sarah Polk, MD, ScM, at the Johns Hopkins Bayview Medical Center has published multiple commentaries that call attention to the crisis in child and adolescent health sparked by draconian immigration policies and that suggest urgent reforms.[13-15]

Another avenue for bringing about change is partnership with public officials. Pediatric health professionals can call public officials with concerns, as well as support health officers and legislators behind the scenes as they investigate. In one case, pediatricians contacted a member of Congress about changes to rules in tae kwon do that put younger adolescents at risk for severe head trauma. The member of Congress then successfully advocated for change.[16]

Some of the most influential advocacy efforts use an "all of the above" approach. An example is B'more for Healthy Babies,[17] a collective impact effort that started in 2009, after headlines announced a spike in infant mortality rates in Baltimore, with enormous disparities in mortality rates between Black and white babies. Since that time, more than 100 groups, including pediatric practices, have joined together to promote safe sleep, discourage tobacco use, recognize the role of racism in producing poor health for mothers and babies, and tackle fundamental inequities facing families across the city. Baltimore's infant mortality rate has since fallen to record lows, with substantial declines in disparities. Recently, city leaders celebrated a 75% decline in infant death in the Upton/Druid Heights neighborhood, the site of the most intense work by B'more for Healthy Babies. The city's health commissioner, pediatrician Letitia Dzirasa, MD, stated, "Our celebration of the record low Black infant mortality rate in Upton/Druid Heights is a testament to the power of collaboration and sustained community investment."[18]

Conclusion

At every point in their careers, pediatric health professionals can work to advance racial equity in their communities. Pediatric residency programs are now required to provide "structured educational experiences that prepare residents for the role of advocate for the health of the children and adolescents within the community."[19] Pediatricians in practice have led campaigns against child poverty,[20] against teen vaping,[21] and for reduced gun violence.[22] Even retired pediatric health professionals can use their time, experience, and community connections to support efforts for change.

If any inspiration is needed, pediatric health professionals need only think of Flint. In an interview with the *Journal of the American Medical Association*, Dr Hanna-Attisha stated:

> *I want to reiterate to the medical community that you have tremendous power and privilege in your voice. When you can address a community issue or a public health crisis, it really is powerful.[23]*

Summary

Pediatric health professionals can bring their knowledge and leadership to expose the impact of racism on child health in their communities. They can work with community partners and others to propose and advocate for effective solutions.

Recommendations

Clinical Practice/Organizations/Systems

● Identify issues in your clinical practice that reflect the adverse consequences of racism and discrimination on child health.

Public Health Policy and Community Advocacy

● Collect and analyze data on these issues to understand their scope and impact.

● Work with families, community leaders, health officials, and others to develop programmatic and policy solutions to these problems.

● Advocate for change, including by helping legislators develop and pass legislation that advances equity and child health.

References

1. Hanna-Attisha M. *What the Eyes Don't See: A Story of Crisis, Resistance, and Hope in an American City.* One World; 2018

2. Hanna-Attisha M, LaChance J, Sadler RC, Champney Schnepp A. Elevated blood lead levels in children associated with the Flint drinking water crisis: a spatial analysis of risk and public health response. *Am J Public Health.* 2016;106(2):283–290 PMID: 26691115 doi: 10.2105/AJPH.2015.303003

3. Doctors urge Flint to switch water after kids' blood tests show lead poisoning. CBS News. September 24, 2015. Accessed February 21, 2023. https://www.cbsnews.com/detroit/news/doctors-urge-flint-to-stop-using-water-from-flint-river-due-to-lead-in-blood

4. Doerfler G. Researcher describes environmental racism in Flint in Klau Center lecture. *Observer.* September 28, 2020. Accessed February 21, 2023. https://ndsmcobserver.com/2020/09/researcher-describes-environmental-racism-in-flint-in-klau-center-lecture

5. Office of the Press Secretary. Fact sheet: federal support for the Flint water crisis response and recovery. News release. White House; May 3, 2016. Accessed February 21, 2023. https://obamawhitehouse.archives.gov/the-press-office/2016/05/03/fact-sheet-federal-support-Flint-water-crisis-response-and-recovery

6. Fact sheet: the Biden-Harris Lead Pipe and Paint Action Plan. News release. White House; December 16, 2021. Accessed February 21, 2023. https://www.whitehouse.gov/briefing-room/statements-releases/2021/12/16/fact-sheet-the-biden-harris-lead-pipe-and-paint-action-plan

7. Cook L. US education: still separate and unequal. *US News & World Report.* January 28, 2015. Accessed February 21, 2023. https://www.usnews.com/news/blogs/data-mine/2015/01/28/us-education-still-separate-and-unequal

8. Spievack N. For people of color, employment disparities start early. *Urban Wire* blog. July 25, 2019. Accessed February 21, 2023. https://www.urban.org/urban-wire/people-color-employment-disparities-start-early

9. Jackson AN, Butler-Barnes ST, Stafford JD, Robinson H, Allen PC. "Can I live": black American adolescent boys' reports of police abuse and the role of religiosity on mental health. *Int J Environ Res Public Health.* 2020;17(12):4330 PMID: 32560418 doi: 10.3390/ijerph17124330

10. The Institute of Medicine Committee for the Study of the Future of Public Health. *The Future of Public Health.* National Academies Press; 1988

11. Bowie L. Baltimore city students have missed almost 1.5 million hours of class time because of inadequate school facilities. *Baltimore Sun.* February 4, 2020. Accessed February 21, 2023. https://www.baltimoresun.com/education/bs-md-ci-school-facilities-jhu-study-20200204-schzujfgozgabbzmsuub7xlfia-story.html

12. DOC4Kids. *Not Safe at Home: How America's Housing Crisis Threatens the Health of Its Children.* Sandel M, Sharfstein J, eds. Boston Medical Center and Children's Hospital; 1998. Accessed February 21, 2023. https://books.google.com/books/about/Not_Safe_at_Home.html?id=1-fZAAAAMAAJ

13. Page KR, Venkataramani M, Beyrer C, Polk S. Undocumented U.S. immigrants and COVID-19. *N Engl J Med.* 2020;382(21):e62 PMID: 32220207 doi: 10.1056/NEJMp2005953

14. Berlin A, Koski-Karell V, Page KR, Polk S. The right and left hands of the state—two patients at risk of deportation. *N Engl J Med.* 2019;381(3):197–201 PMID: 31314963 doi: 10.1056/NEJMp1811607

15. Polk S, Richards S, Hernando MA, Moon M, Sharfstein J. Children as pawns of US immigration policy. *J Appl Res Child.* 2019;10(1). Accessed February 21, 2023. https://digitalcommons.library.tmc.edu/childrenatrisk/vol10/iss1/1

16. Associated Press. Officials worry about athlete head trauma. ESPN. May 20, 2004. Accessed February 21, 2023. https://www.espn.com/olympics/news/story?id=1805836

17. Baltimore City Health Department. B'more for Healthy Babies. Accessed February 21, 2023. https://health.baltimorecity.gov/maternal-and-child-health/bmore-healthy-babies

18. Scott BM. Mayor, health department and partners celebrate reduction of infant mortality rate in Upton/Druid Heights neighborhood through work of B'more for Healthy Babies. News release. City of Baltimore; June 15, 2021. Accessed February 21, 2023. https://mayor.baltimorecity.gov/news/press-releases/2021-06-15-mayor-health-department-and-partners-celebrate-reduction-infant

19. Chamberlain LJ, Sanders LM, Takayama JI. Child advocacy training: curriculum outcomes and resident satisfaction. *Arch Pediatr Adolesc Med.* 2005;159(9):842–847 PMID: 16143743 doi: 10.1001/archpedi.159.9.842

20. Plax K, Donnelly J, Federico SG, Brock L, Kaczorowski JM. An essential role for pediatricians: becoming child poverty change agents for a lifetime. *Acad Pediatr.* 2016;16(3)(suppl):S147–S154 PMID: 27044693 doi: 10.1016/j.acap.2016.01.009

21. Tomassi A. Yale pediatricians named "e-cigarette champions" by CT-AAP. Yale School of Medicine. May 12, 2021. Accessed February 21, 2023. https://medicine.yale.edu/news-article/yale-pediatricians-named-e-cigarette-champions-by-ct-aap

22. Fox M. Pediatricians to lobby Congress for gun control laws. NBC News. April 9, 2018. Accessed February 21, 2023. https://www.nbcnews.com/health/health-news/pediatricians-lobby-congress-gun-control-laws-n864116

23. Abbasi J. Lead, mistrust, and trauma—whistleblowing pediatrician discusses the legacy of Flint's water crisis. *JAMA.* 2021;325(21):2136–2139 PMID: 33978707 doi: 10.1001/jama.2021.2314

CHAPTER 35

Conclusion

Maria Trent, MD, MPH; Danielle G. Dooley, MD, MPhil;
and Jacqueline Dougé, MD, MPH

"Not everything that is faced can be changed, but nothing can be changed until it is faced." The words of James Baldwin resonate deeply with the work needed to dismantle structural racism and its impact on the health and well-being of infants, children, adolescents, and young adults. The American Academy of Pediatrics has taken on this work, ready to support pediatric health professionals as we embrace the responsibility to advocate for all infants, children, adolescents, and young adults, as well as their families.

We recognize that children, adolescents, and families can face health disparities solely because of their identity. Compounding the well-documented history of discrimination, the ongoing circumstances of it—along with the multitude of policies and laws that are discriminatory and threaten what young people can be taught or read, what clinical services young people can receive, and even if they can safely exist in all environments—continue to be a challenge. Despite these setbacks, we live in a heterogeneous and global society, and the pediatric populations we serve are the most diverse in our nation's history. There is often a sense that we have gone back in time, and many health professionals may feel weary and lean into apathy, but remaining forward-looking is central to our scope of practice. We must not give up hope.

Pediatric health professionals are trusted champions for child health, and, in this role, we address barriers that impede children from obtaining optimal health. When we acknowledge that racism is woven into the fabric of our society, structural racism becomes a central barrier we must overcome to optimize the environments in which children live, play, and learn. As health professionals, we tackle other barriers to optimal health when we screen for and address adverse childhood experiences and social determinants of physical and mental health. Ignoring the impact of racism on child, adolescent, and parental/caregiver well-being, however, prevents us from fully comprehending and addressing our children's identities, experiences, and contexts.

To better understand the effect of racism on these issues, we first delved into the social determinants of health and explored how racism drives health inequities. Recognizing that children at different developmental stages experience and understand racism differently is vital in our efforts to address structural racism. We discussed the developmental stages that children learn about racial and ethnic identities. Although it is true that infants can detect physical differences across individuals, the pediatric health professional must understand that adults shape the meaning of those observations and how children internalize adult cues as they develop. Adolescents are often overlooked in these discussions but have been shown to shoulder a more significant burden of managing differences as their intersectional factors collide during this critical phase to shape identity development. Understanding how these socially constructed categories are further compounded by gender and sexuality will allow us to provide better anticipatory guidance as crucial life decisions, including risk management, are made during this key period in the life course. Intersectional factors on the experience of racism, such as gender and sexuality, can become complicated when discrimination is layered on the developing youth within their families and the larger world, leading to an identity crisis with concurrent mental health challenges.

A misconception persists that the work to address racism excludes white children, as they are often not considered part of the diversity spectrum. The homogeny of whiteness often yields substantial political power, but white children bring experiences of language, religion, and culture that shaped their upbringing and interactions with others. Those raised in multicultural communities with diverse peer and friend groups are more successful academically and socially as teenagers and in the workplace as adults. The chapter on supporting white children and adolescents to embrace diversity (Chapter 23) was not only unique but critically important, as we offered ideas regarding their development and evolving role as allies for their minoritized peers. We also provided information to support children of other racial/Multiracial and ethnic identities and immigration status. We offered guidance on challenging long-held negative stereotypes and assumptions that hinder equitable access to resources, including health care.

Last, we shared ways for health professionals to realistically get started and operationalize the tools and resources in the office setting. Scenarios were shared, demonstrating how health professionals can talk with families about race and racism and help families raise children to be resisters against racism, an important skill to help build resilience. Additionally, we highlighted clinical practice and how engagement with community partners can address the social, educational, political, economic, environmental, and cultural determinants of child and adolescent health, including steps to transform organizations and systems, policy and practice, and the role of advocacy.

To dismantle the impact of systemic racism on child and adolescent health, we must acknowledge our history. We must also recognize the frustration and disproportionate burden experienced by minoritized health professionals often asked to lead problem-solving with limited support from colleagues and institutions. In all the movements that have carried the arc of justice forward in the United States, there have been allies who are ready to stand with minoritized people, contribute to social change, unlearn harm, and help transform systems of inequity into systems of equity. These individuals and groups proactively remove themselves from places of privilege and comfort to those of calculated risk because they are intuitive about our future world and the need to advance civil rights, women's rights, LGBTQ+ rights, and reproductive justice. This history serves as evidence of the power of collective action. In pediatric health, prevention is critical to honor our oath to "do no harm," as our approach has always been that growth and change in our populations are possible and necessary for them to meet the milestones to successfully launch as young adults.

Our next steps require collective action, with individual patients and families in practice and as an interdisciplinary workforce advocating for a different health and societal structure for our patients. By implementing intentional cross-sector partnerships, advocating for legislative and policy changes, and leading clinical, organizational, and systemic changes in health care, we can begin to untangle the threads of racism that are strangling youth development and stagnating society. Ultimately, we must step outside our examination rooms, practices, and offices and work within our communities, school boards, and governments to ensure a future in which every child thrives.

Index

C

Centers for Disease Control and Prevention, 25, 215

Character, as developmental factor, 192*b*

Childhood innocence, 163

Child welfare system, 229

Climate change, 136

Collaboration for health equity, 5

"Collective forgetting," 171–172

Color-blind casting, 187

Color-blind parenting, 163

Color-conscious casting, 187

Color-conscious racial messages, 170

Colorism, 64*b*

Competence, as developmental factor, 192*b*

Confidence, as developmental factor, 192*b*

Connection, as developmental factor, 192*b*, 193, 194–195*t*

Contraception. *See* Reproductive justice

Contribution, as developmental factor, 192*b*

Control, as developmental factor, 192*b*

Conversations with white children and adolescents about racism

addressing racism in early childhood, 170

introduction to, 169–170

observations and interactions in middle childhood, 170–171

power of actions and modeling behavior throughout childhood and, 171–172

recommendations on, 172–173

Coping, as developmental factor, 192*b*

COVID-19 pandemic

inequities highlighted during, 3, 109

media use during, 185

Native American/Alaska Native (AI/AN) populations during, 46

opportunity youth during, 227

poverty during, 10

racial trauma during, 176

Critical consciousness, as developmental factor, 192*b*, 196

Cultural competency, 83

Culturally congruent mentoring, 157

Culturally congruent strategies

current demographics of the pediatric health workforce and, 153, 155*t*

Enhancing Mentoring, 157–159, 158*f*

implicit bias and, 156

introduction to, 153, 154*b*

recommendations on, 159–160

structural and institutional racism in medical education and, 156–157

Cultural socialization, 27

Culture, defined, 154*b*

Culture of respect, 213–214

D

Data, race and ethnicity, 4

Dawes Act of 1887, 103

Deferred Action for Childhood Arrivals, 64

Demographic forms, 40–41

Developmental stages when talking about race, 206–207

Differential offending, 127–129, 128–129*t*, 128*f*

Differential treatment, 127–129, 128–129*t*, 128*f*

Digital literacy, 187–188

Disconnected youth, 227. *See also* Opportunity youth

Discrimination, 25, 64*b*

impact on adolescents, 33–34

policies on, 214

protecting youth against, 27, 28*t*

reporting of, 215–216

training on, 214–215

Diversity management, 213–216

Drowning

rates of, 101

role of inequity and racism in, 101–103

E

Early childhood education (ECE), 111

Early intervention (EI), 76

Education

advocacy through, 246

benefits of high-quality, 109–110

bias in, 17, 17*t*

early childhood (ECE), 111

extracurricular activities and, 112

gifted and talented programs, 112